KU-016-080

ACKNOWLEDGEMENTS

I would like to thank everyone who has contributed their thoughts, expertise and advice as well as words of encouragement. Some are mentioned individually below but many others are not and to you all I owe a huge debt of gratitude. Special thanks particularly to the army of proofreaders who gave of their time freely and whose feedback enabled the book to grow and develop. A special mention goes out to David French and the Gold Duke of Edinburgh pupils from Tomlinscote School & Sixth Form College and Wavell's Butchers in Llanrug for their contribution to the 'wounds' section.

I wish to express my sincere gratitude to those who kindly contributed to the 'Real Life Stories' that appear throughout the book. I know for some it meant revisiting particularly difficult memories and feelings which took great effort and courage. Their first-hand accounts provide a unique insight from the casualty's perspective and greatly enhance the main text.

In the field of grammar thank you to Anna Cosslett, Alan Gale, and Mandi Shipton for their guidance and particular thanks to Anna who saw me through all five years of the book's development and whose endless enthusiasm, especially during the harder stages of the process, drove me on.

Although first aid is **not** medicine I would like to thank the following people for their professional opinions, suggestions and guidance.

Professor Chris Imray (PhD, FRCS, FRCP, Dip Mount. Med, Consultant Vascular and Endovascular Surgeon, Warwick Medical School, UHCW NHS Trust Coventry, CV2 2DX, and UK frostbite advice team member).

Professor David A Warrell (Emeritus Professor of Tropical Medicine and Honorary Fellow of St Cross College, University of Oxford).

Lt Col RJ Russell (Head, Academic Department of Military Emergency Medicine, Royal Centre for Defense Medicine. Hon Senior Lecturer Military Emergency Medicine, University of Birmingham).

Dr Caroline Leech (Consultant in Emergency Medicine & Pre-hospital Care).

Dr David Hillebrandt (Vice president UIAA Medcom, International Society of Mountain Medicine, Hon Medical advisor to BMC, and UK frostbite advice team member).

Dr Ian Johnson (Anaesthesia /ICU medicine, Ysbyty Gwynedd)

Dr Jennie Ormerod (Consultant Clinical Psychologist, Humber Traumatic Stress Service).

Dr John Ellerton (Chairman of the Mountain Rescue (England and Wales) Medical Sub Committee, Team Doctor for Patterdale Mountain Rescue).

Dr John Glynne Andrew (Trauma and Orthopaedic Surgeon, Medical Officer for Ogwen Valley Mountain Rescue Team).

Dr Linda Dykes (FCEM Consultant in Emergency Medicine, Director of the Ysbyty Gwynedd Mountain Medicine Project).

Dr Pauline Cutting (FCEM retired, Consultant in Emergency Medicine, Ysbyty Gwynedd).

Dr Steve Rowe (Anaesthetist, Medical Officer Edale Mountain Rescue Team, Doctor with Yorkshire Air Ambulance).

Dr William Sutcliff (Anaesthetist, Medical Officer Llanberis Mountain Rescue Team).

Master Aircrewman Richard Taylor QGM cfs (RAF Search and Rescue Winchman Paramedic).

Paramedic Steven Pile (Paramedic with the Welsh Ambulance Service).

Paramedic Harold Burrows MBE (Medical officer for the North Wales Mountain Rescue Association (NWMRA), Paramedic and Training officer for Gwent Ambulance Service (retired), Member of North East Wales Search and Rescue Team, Search and Rescue Dog Handler).

Nurse Phil Benbow (Psychiatric nurse, Chairman of the North Wales Mountain Rescue Association (NWMRA), team member and secretary of Llanberis Mountain Rescue Team and Search and Rescue Dog Association Member).

And finally to my husband Brian whose entertaining words of encouragement and his patience deserve a bigger thank you than I am able to express here.

ABOUT THE AUTHOR

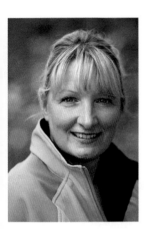

Katherine is a qualified Specialist Physical Education teacher and currently runs Active First Aid Training, delivering Rescue Emergency Care certified courses throughout the UK. Having lived in Snowdonia for over twenty-five years she is passionate about mountaineering. In 2000 Katherine became a member of the Llanberis Mountain Rescue Team and since then has attended over 350 rescue incidents. She holds the Mountain Rescue Councils Casualty Care first aid certificate as well as the Emergency Care in Mountain Rescue (Advanced) certificate. Katherine spent a number of years as the chair of the rescue team's Medical Sub-committee and holds the Queen's Golden Jubilee Medal for her services to mountain rescue.

Details of Katherine's Active First Aid Training courses can be found at **www.activefirstaid.co.uk**

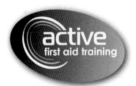

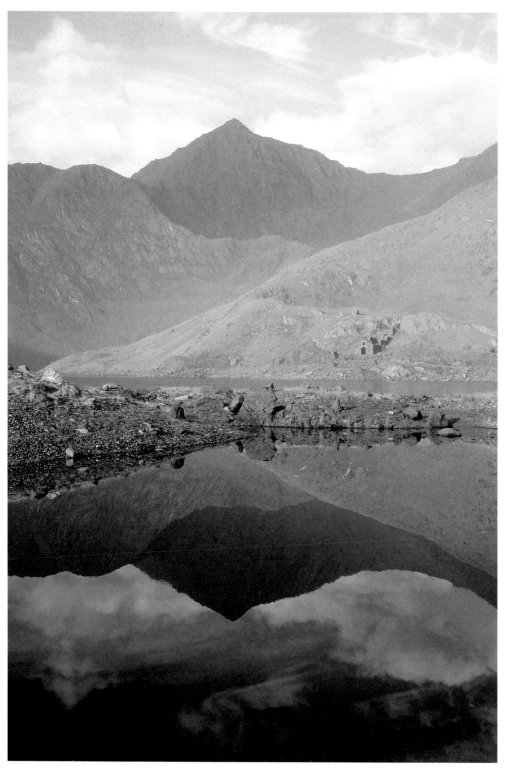

Snowdon from Llyn Llydaw.

Photo: Brian Wills

INTRODUCTION

The great outdoors provides us with a playground and, for some, a place of work. Whether you are a walker, paraglider, orienteer, climber, horse rider, mountain biker or fell runner, all outdoor activities carry inherent risks and dangers. In fact, seeking and controlling those risks can, for some, be a part of the whole enjoyment. Because of this, there has to be an acceptance that injury could be a consequence of taking part in such activities. We must therefore be prepared to have to deal with an accident (or some form of medical problem) possibly in an isolated, inaccessible or even hostile environment.

In an urban setting we rely on ambulance crews, paramedics, doctors and nurses to provide assistance and medical care when things go wrong. This usually means the average person can get away with knowing surprisingly little first aid, but remain fairly safe on a day to day basis. However, once you enter the remote setting, your minimal first aid knowledge and skills may suddenly feel inadequate.

The remote setting

Broadly speaking, the term 'remote' refers to a location that is some distance away from civilisation, where if medical assistance is required, it could be some time before that help arrives and the casualty is evacuated to hospital. Although it is true to say a farm house situated in the far corners of the Scottish Highlands could be viewed as remote, in the context of this book the remote setting refers specifically to an outdoor location away from immediate help and assistance.

First aid in the remote setting

Remote first aid is very different from its urban counterpart in three distinct areas. First, medical help can be some considerable distance away, and because of this, time spent with the casualty is extended and an element of 'nursing' becomes an important part of the treatment. (Throughout the book the term 'casualty' has been used to describe someone who is in need of first aid.)

Tied in with this is the concept of casualty evacuation – removing a casualty from the remote setting – by either self-evacuation or through the rescue services. Self-evacuation is when the first aider, or casualty, takes care of the whole process. A rescue evacuation, on the other hand, involves staying where you are, insulating the casualty from the ground, providing shelter and summoning medical help to your location. In the UK this is provided by the Mountain Rescue Service, who can be reached by dialling 999 or 112, asking for **police** and then requesting **mountain rescue.**

The second difference is the outdoor environment itself: we need to consider not only the position of the casualty, but also the prevailing weather conditions. In some instances, the casualty can come to rest in extremely dangerous or awkward places, such as on steep ground or head first in a narrow gully. The prevailing weather conditions can make administering first aid quite challenging, as well as limiting which rescue resources can be used (i.e. a helicopter) and the speed with which rescue teams on foot can reach you.

Finally there may be a limited first aid kit available; you will only have whatever you choose to carry. This means that on occasions you will need to improvise and, at times, apply a little imagination. Successful improvisation relies on a sound understanding of the principles behind the first aid given. To adapt equipment or kit effectively you will need to ask yourself, "What is it I am trying to achieve, and what have I got to help me do that?"

Due to these three unique aspects of remote first aid, some of the information presented here may differ from first aid books and courses geared towards the urban environment. The treatments suggested are based on the premise that medical help is some considerable time away; therefore a number of procedures presented should not be attempted if medical assistance is expected to arrive quickly.

This book provides an invaluable insight into the challenges of first aid in the outdoor environment. Although many health professionals have been consulted during its development (the vast majority of whom have experience of applying their clinical skills in the remote setting) it is important to emphasise that the contents cover basic first aid and not remote medicine.

Health professionals who work in the urban environment may find the information presented rather different from what is normally advocated in a conventional clinical setting.

Although an essential resource, this book should not be used as a substitute for attending a structured first aid course geared towards the outdoor environment delivered by a knowledgeable and experienced instructor. First aid skills need to be practised in an environment which allows you to safely develop judgement and casualty-handling before doing it for real. In the remote setting you may be placed in a situation where you have to treat injuries and medical conditions which you would not normally be expected to deal with when an ambulance is only a few minutes away.

Chris and his mate Brian are descending the track from the summit. They've had a long day and the weather has not been kind, plus to cap it all it's getting dark. On the steep rocky section at the top of the track Chris trips and falls over the edge and out of sight. Brian, horrified, comes running down and around a rocky outcrop to see Chris holding what is obviously a broken leg shouting "HELP ME!" Brian stares in disbelief. His mobile is out of signal and it's a good hour's walk to get help.

Apart from panicking, what might you do in Brian's place?

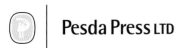

For details of all the outdoor and adventure sport
books available from Pesda Press visit

www.pesdapress.com

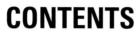

CONTENTS

It's not Rocket science ...

Keep them breathing.

Stop them bleeding.

Keep them warm.

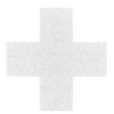

1. DEALING WITH A CONSCIOUS CASUALTY

As a first aider it is quite normal to feel a little apprehensive when the time comes for you to put your training into action. However, you must try to stay calm and take control of the situation. This chapter presents you with a systematic approach, called a **remote casualty assessment**, which gives you a clear plan of action and helps guide you to do the right things in the right order.

The conscious casualty

Casualties can be frightened, upset, confused or even on occasions aggressive; it can be quite a challenge to know how to handle them! Your experience and ability to communicate clearly, in a calm and sensitive way, are important. Offering reassurance and support are essential tools for the first aider in any environment, but particularly so in the remote setting when help can be a long way away. Don't underestimate the importance of a simple act such as holding a casualty's hand or placing your hand on their shoulder. Good communication and a confident, but compassionate approach are often as important as your first aid treatment. You need to establish a rapport and build trust with the casualty quickly.

Gaining consent

You must ask the casualty's permission to help them – you need to gain their consent. Despite the fact that they may clearly need first aid, it is within their rights to refuse. Gently reassure them and explain why you feel they need your help. However, if they continue to refuse and in your opinion they are of 'sound mind' and able to make a rational decision then you must back away.

If you step forward to assist and the casualty agrees then you have a 'duty of care' to that person to use your first aid knowledge and skills in a sensible and responsible way. Work within the boundaries of what you have been trained to do and feel confident doing; take care not to cause further harm.

Care of casualty's possessions

If possible, keep the casualty's belongings together and with them. If summoning help from mountain rescue, ensure they are made aware of rucksacks, climbing kit, bike, etc. In the event of the casualty being airlifted by helicopter, their belongings may go with them, or simply left for the casualty's friends or mountain rescue to sort out. If you end up with a casualty's belongings, and you don't know them, take the possessions to the closest mountain rescue base, or police station.

Personal possessions may on occasions include the casualty's pet – for example a dog, or horse. If possible, try to keep the animal close or in sight of the casualty; if they are taken away, the casualty can become extremely agitated and upset. However, be aware of the necessary safety issues should a rescue helicopter be first on scene.

Remote casualty assessment: conscious

Casualties do not always require a full detailed and lengthy assessment; a common-sense approach will be needed. For example, a casualty who cuts their hand on a knife while slicing an apple at lunch would probably not require a secondary survey. If, however, the cut hand is from falling off a horse while jumping a gate, there is the likelihood of further injuries and a full and thorough assessment would be both appropriate and essential.

Undertaking a casualty assessment in the outdoors can be difficult. You may find yourself on a narrow ledge in the dark, battling with severe weather conditions with hands that are cold, wet and numb, with a casualty wrapped up in several layers of clothing in an awkward location! You may find doing even the simplest of first aid procedures quite challenging.

The following casualty assessment is geared towards the remote environment; therefore the sequence, considerations and actions differ from the common urban approach.

The assessment is divided into four levels:

1. Scene survey.

2. Initial assessment including a Primary survey.

3. Secondary survey.

4. Continue the activity or Evacuate the casualty.

1	**Scene survey** Danger

2	**Initial assessment** Level of response **Primary survey** Check **A**irway Check **B**reathing Check **C**irculation

3	**Secondary survey** Conscious casualty with injury and/or medical condition

4	**Continue the activity**	**Evacuate the casualty**

Self-evacuation

Dial 999/112
Request police – then
ask for mountain rescue

1. Scene survey

The scene survey involves rapidly assessing any actual or potential dangers to yourself, the casualty (and others), and forming some initial impressions about what has happened.

1   **Scene survey**
Danger
What has happened?

2   **Initial assessment**
Level of response

Primary survey
Check **A**irway
Check **B**reathing
Check **C**irculation

3   **Secondary survey**
Conscious casualty with injury
and/or medical condition

4   **Continue the activity**   **Evacuate the casualty**

Self-evacuation   Dial 999/112
Request police – then
ask for mountain rescue

Danger

Every incident will be different but the emphasis remains the same, **your safety must come first**. In the remote setting, dangers may include such things as steep terrain, rock falls, flooding, lightning strikes and falling trees. In winter, these can also include the risk of falling ice, reckless skiers or snowboarders, or avalanches. Take the time to check for any dangers before you approach; rushing in without thinking could simply add to the list of casualties.

If the scene is safe, but you identify a potential hazard – remember the outdoor setting can be dynamic and challenging to control – ask a member of your group, or a helpful bystander, to monitor the possible danger and alert you if necessary.

Having decided to approach the scene of an incident, take the time to work out the least dangerous route. When you reach the casualty (or if you were with the casualty when the incident happened) you will need to quickly decide if it is safe for you to remain where you are or to move to a less dangerous location (see the chapter on **Moving and Carrying a Casualty**).

What has happened?

As you approach the scene, try to form an immediate impression about what is going on. This could be an accident which has resulted in an injury, or perhaps someone who is feeling unwell; or both.

Mechanisms of injury

With an accident it is important to establish what exactly happened – the 'mechanisms of injury'. You may have seen the incident or there may be bystanders who witnessed it. Useful questions (depending on what happened) may include:

"When did this happen and has the casualty moved since?"

"Was the casualty wearing a helmet?"

"How far did they fall?"

If they fell "did they go head first, feet first, onto an outstretched hand?"

"Were they conscious throughout?"

Establishing the mechanisms of injury will guide you towards identifying the potential for certain types of injuries and on occasions highlight the possibility of a spinal injury – which may affect how you manage the airway in the next stage. For a suspected spinal injury ask yourself "could they have hurt their neck or back?" If the answer is "maybe", then as you approach, tell the casualty to stay completely still and not move.

Multiple casualties

(see the chapter on **Multiple Casualty Incidents: Triage***).*

Quickly establish how many people are in need of first aid; if necessary look for bystanders who may be able to provide this information. If there is more than one person, quickly find out which casualties need to be treated first.

Nature of the medical condition

Medical conditions pose a different challenge. Your initial impressions will guide you towards establishing what is causing the person to feel unwell and whether this is a known chronic (long-term) condition which they normally manage themselves.

2. Initial assessment – primary survey

After the **scene survey,** move on to the **initial assessment**. Establish the casualty's **level of response** (are they conscious or unconscious) and if appropriate, shout for help from other bystanders. Then complete a **primary survey**, including checks to the **A**irway, **B**reathing and **C**irculation.

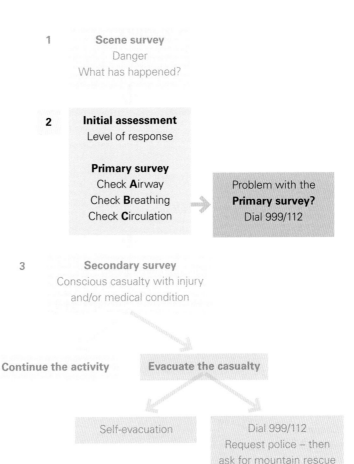

1   **Scene survey**
Danger
What has happened?

2   **Initial assessment**
Level of response

Primary survey
Check **A**irway
Check **B**reathing
Check **C**irculation

Problem with the
Primary survey?
Dial 999/112

3   **Secondary survey**
Conscious casualty with injury
and/or medical condition

4   **Continue the activity**   **Evacuate the casualty**

Self-evacuation

Dial 999/112
Request police – then
ask for mountain rescue

Level of response (AVPU)

Your initial task is to find out if the casualty is conscious or not; this is done using a scale called **AVPU** (**A**lert, **V**oice, **P**ain or **U**nresponsive). Look at them as you approach, do they look conscious? Ask them a question such as "Are you ok?". The conscious casualty will be **A**lert (the **A** of **AVPU**) and respond to your questions. Make eye contact with them and if they are unknown to you introduce yourself; ask them their name, what happened and whether you can help. If they fail to respond then gently squeeze their shoulder; if there is still no response, they are unconscious (**VPU** of **AVPU**). Assessing the unconscious casualty is covered in the following chapter.

CONSCIOUS CASUALTY = ALERT

The conscious casualty is **alert**, speaks clearly and responds to questions. They spontaneously open their eyes when you approach, react to your voice (though they may be confused) and appear to be aware of, and react to, their environment.

Depending on the situation (for example if you come upon casualty while out walking alone), consider shouting for help from anyone who might hear you.

The primary survey – ABC

The primary survey – **A**irway, **B**reathing, and **C**irculation – is part of your rapid initial assessment and guides you towards detecting any life-threatening conditions which need your immediate attention. If the casualty is conscious and talking, this survey may be completed reasonably quickly.

Check airway

Your initial concern is with the airway, which must be open and clear. A casualty who is conscious (alert) and speaking has an open and clear airway. A number of conditions may cause problems with the airway; including choking and anaphylactic shock (see the chapter on **Breathing Problems**). If the mechanisms of injury give you cause to suspect that the casualty may have an injury to the neck, or they are complaining of pain in the neck or back, you should suspect a possible spine or back injury. Tell the casualty not to move. If you are on your own, ask them to stay still while you continue with your assessment; if another person is available, ask them to take hold of the head in the neutral position and keep it completely still (see the chapter on **Spine and Back Injuries**).

Check breathing

The next step is to make sure the casualty is breathing normally. The conscious casualty who is talking will be breathing. If they are able to speak in clear unhurried sentences, there is unlikely to be a major breathing problem. If, however, their words are hurried and in short 'half' sentences or they are only able to grunt or make noises, they are having breathing difficulties. This could be due to either an injury or medical condition (see the chapter on **Breathing Problems**).

Check circulation

Your priority here is to identify any life-threatening bleeding and, if it is external and leaking out, stop it! For internal bleeding there is often very little you can do directly other than identify its presence and urgently summon help. Life-threatening bleeding, whether external or internal, causes a casualty to go into shock and you should be familiar with how to recognise and treat both (see the chapter on **Life-threatening Bleeding and Shock**).

After checking for and stopping any external life-threatening bleeding you should also include an assessment of the casualty's skin colour; for example, have they turned pale or blue? Check their mental status – are they anxious, agitated, confused or drowsy? If you are able to, take a pulse (see the section below on **Monitoring vital signs**).

Problems in the primary survey

Any problems found in your **ABC** check are usually serious. Ask a member of your party, or a bystander, to urgently call for help – this is an **emergency**. To call out mountain rescue dial 999 (or 112), request **police**, then ask for **mountain rescue**; pass on the details of the incident, providing as much information as possible. Make it clear you have a potentially life-threatening emergency. For information on calling out mountain rescue and what to do when they arrive (see the chapter on **Working with Rescue Services**).

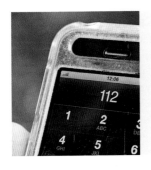

CALLING THE EMERGENCY SERVICES 999 OR 112

Many countries have a single emergency telephone number that allows the caller to summon help from the emergency services – police, fire or ambulance. In the 1990s a common European emergency number was created – 112 – which can be used alongside all other emergency numbers. Therefore in the UK if you require an emergency service you can call either 999 or 112.

3. The secondary survey

This part of your casualty assessment involves dealing with the injury or medical condition, and where appropriate, undertaking a more detailed head-to-toe examination to find any other problems which may not be as obvious. A simple way to remember how to approach your secondary survey is to use the mnemonic **SAMPLE**.

*The **SAMPLE** mnemonic does not have to be undertaken in this specific order. In fact **E** – **E**vents; what happened? – is probably going to be one of the first things you ask, followed closely by an assessment of **S** (**S**igns and **S**ymptoms).*

LOOK OUT FOR

S – Signs and symptoms.

A – Allergies.

M – Medications.

P – Previous medical history.

L – Last meal.

E – Events; what happened?

WHAT TO DO

Signs and symptoms: Signs are things you can see or feel such as bleeding, bruising, swelling, etc. Symptoms are experienced by the casualty, who may describe them to you, for example being in pain.

Allergies: Is the casualty allergic to anything such as medications, latex, etc?

Medication: Is the casualty taking either prescription or over the counter drugs? If yes, write down what, how often and how much they take (also whether they have taken any on that day).

Previous medical history: There may be a past injury or medical condition that could account for, or contribute to, the current situation. It is important to note if the casualty has any other medical conditions such as pregnancy, asthma, diabetes or heart problems even if this may not currently be causing any concern.

Last meal: Make a note of the time they last ate or drank.

Events: Establish a clear picture of what happened, including how the casualty was behaving leading up to, or just before, the incident.

1   **Scene survey**
Danger
What has happened?

2   **Initial assessment**
Level of response

Primary survey
Check **A**irway
Check **B**reathing
Check **C**irculation

Problem with the
Primary survey?
Dial 999/112

3   **Secondary survey**
Conscious casualty with injury
and/or medical condition

Take a history – S A M P L E
Injury?
Treat any injuries
Perform a head-to-toe if
appropriate
Medical conditions?
What's the problem?
Is there a past history of this
problem?
Are they, or you, carrying any
medication?
Take vital signs

4   Continue the activity   **Evacuate the casualty**

Self-evacuation

Dial 999/112
Request police – then
ask for mountain
rescue

The injured casualty

Kneel down to the casualty's height, make eye contact and listen carefully to what they are saying; avoid the temptation to interrupt. Try to adopt a calm and confident approach, keeping your sentences short and simple, and don't rush. Explain what you think is wrong and how you plan to treat them; give options and if possible, get them involved in their own treatment.

The signs and symptoms will guide you towards their complaint and your initial treatment will be focused there. It is always worth asking if they are hurting anywhere else, to establish the likelihood of another injury else-where. If the casualty says they are fine, but you suspect there might be other injuries the casualty is not aware of, it may be appropriate to suggest you give them a quick check over (head-to-toe examination).

The head-to-toe examination

Throughout your examination ask the casualty if they feel any pain or discomfort.

Examining a casualty can be very challenging in the outdoor environment; you may need to loosen, open, remove or even cut away clothing. Be mind-ful of the environment you are in, especially when cutting away clothing as this may increase the risk of hypothermia. Ideally, the examination should be done under a **group shelter** (a big windproof bag that resembles the outside of a tent and allows people to gather underneath) which will provide you and the casualty with both privacy and some protection from the ele-ments. Once treatment is complete consider putting clothes back on. Cut clothing can be taped or pinned back in place.

Head

Without moving the head run your hands carefully over the scalp. Do not interfere with any obviously clotting wounds – simply feel for active bleeding, swelling, lumps or depressions (which may indicate a fracture). Check for any fluid leak-ing out of the ears or nose (this can vary from clear to brown/red in appearance). This leaking fluid is an indicator of a fractured skull.

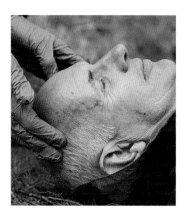

Face

Note the skin colour and temperature; is the casualty pale, blue, or grey? Do they feel cold and clammy, or hot and dry? Look for wounds, swelling or bruising.

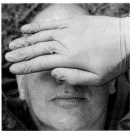

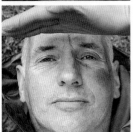

Eyes

Remove glasses. Check the pupils (the black part). They should be the same size and react similarly to light. To test this, place your hand over the eyes to block out the light then quickly take it away; you should notice both pupils becoming smaller as you re-introduce the light. If in the dark use a pen light or something similar. Note any bleeding into the white of the eyes, or any other damage including black eyes (panda eyes).

Mouth

Smell the breath and note anything unusual such as chemical smell, alcohol etc. Note any damage to the teeth, and wounds or burns (including black soot marks) around the mouth.

Neck

Check the front and back of the neck for wounds and bruising. Feel down the spine from the bottom of the skull to the start of the shoulders for any irregularity, swelling, deformity or tenderness. Be cautious if the casualty complains of any pain down the spine and treat as for a spinal injury.

Shoulders, arms, hands and fingers

Feel along the collar bones, shoulders, upper arms, elbows, hands and fingers. Compare one side to the other. Note any pain, tenderness, swelling or deformity. Ask the casualty to move the joints by bending and straightening them. Check for any change in sensation in the arms and hands; test loss of strength by asking them to squeeze your fingers and compare one side to the other.

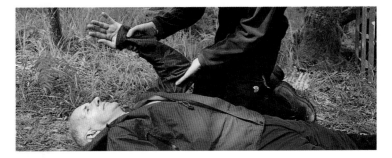

Chest

Ask the casualty to take a deep breath and watch to make sure the chest expands the same on both sides. Note if this causes pain or takes effort. Ask if they are aware of any unusual sensations when breathing. Place both hands flat on the rib cage and gently press to check for pain or tenderness.

If appropriate, check the skin for any wounds, bruising, imprint marks from clothing or equipment.

Abdomen

Gently feel the abdomen for any pain, tenderness or rigidity, indicating possible internal bleeding (rigidity is a late sign). Check the four areas; left and right above the navel and the same below. Check the skin for any wounds, bruising, patterns from clothing or equipment, such as climbing harness, imprinted on the skin.

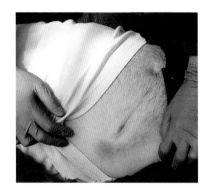

Back and spine

Your assessment of the spine and back will depend on how the casualty is positioned. If they are on their front or side it may be straightforward. If they are lying on their back ask if they have any pain and if possible place your hand under the hollow in the lower part of the back and check for any pain, swelling or tenderness there. If you suspect a spinal injury, treat as if it is.

Pelvis

Do **not** push down on the pelvis. Your assessment should **only** involve establishing the mechanisms of injury (which may indicate the possibility of a pelvic injury) and the casualty's symptoms. Look for signs of incontinence and any obvious bleeding wounds to the skin. If you suspect a pelvic fracture, treat as if it is.

Legs and feet

Look at the legs and note any obvious deformity and wounds. Feel for bleeding, swelling, tenderness or deformity by running your hands down each leg, comparing one side to the other. Ask the casualty if they are able to bend and straighten the joints at the hip, knee and ankle, and ask the casualty to wiggle their toes. Note any changes in circulation and sensation.

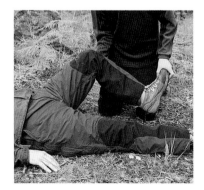

The casualty with a medical condition

A casualty who is unwell could be complaining of a pre-existing medical condition, or it could be the first time they have felt this way. Use your **P**revious medical history assessment (**SAMPLE**) to establish if this is the case.

With a pre-existing condition they may be carrying medication related to their complaint. Make a note of the medication, the amount and time taken and then monitor the casualty for improvement. Understand that the casualty may know what treatment they need; and be guided by them as to whether their symptoms are normal or not.

Alternatively, this may be a new medical condition which they have never experienced before. It is important to develop a basic understanding of the more common medical conditions, such as heart attack, asthma, etc. so that you can recognise the signs and symptoms and identify when a casualty is in need of urgent evacuation to hospital.

Monitoring vital signs

Recording accurate vital signs is important. They give you (and if necessary the rescuers) a set of baseline observations and potentially help you to identify any problems. When monitored they may also help detect any changes in the casualty's condition. There are five basic vital signs.

LOOK OUT FOR

Level of response – AVPU.

Breathing.

Pulse.

Skin colour.

Temperature.

Your findings should be written down preferably on a **casualty report form** (see the chaper on **Outdoor First Aid Kits** for an example) or a note pad.

Level of response – AVPU

An assessment of the casualty's level of response – conscious or unconscious – is undertaken during the initial assessment. The conscious casualty is **A**lert (the **A** of **AVPU**). During the monitoring phase you need to record this on your **casualty report form** or note pad by using the letter that corresponds to their level of response – **A** indicates the casualty is **A**lert and conscious. A score of **V, P** or **U** indicate the casualty is unconscious and is dealt with in the following chapter.

Breathing

Consider the casualty's breathing in relation to rate; the number of breaths in one minute, the rhythm (regular, irregular – does their breathing mimic yours?), and sounds (noiseless, wheezing, gasping). If an adult casualty is breathing less than 10, or more than 30 times in a minute, this is ineffective and is a cause for concern. Remember that children have different breathing to adults (see table).

Photo: Katherine Wills

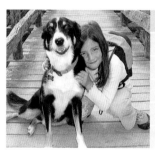

Age (years)	Breaths per minute
less than 1	30–40
1–2	25–35
2–5	25–30
5–12	20–25
more than 12 years	12–20

Taking a pulse

A pulse is basically an artery expanding then contracting with the surge of blood from each heartbeat; they can be notoriously difficult to find, especially in the outdoors. At a basic first level a pulse should only be taken on a casualty who is breathing; and **never** used as an indicator to start resuscitation (the decision to start resuscitation is based on whether a casualty is breathing normally or not).

Pulses are usually taken at the wrist and neck. Always use your fingers, not your thumb (as you have a strong pulse in your thumb). Press gently over the artery against the skin and then record the rate (number of beats in a minute), strength (whether it's strong or weak) and rhythm (if it's regular or irregular).

Neck pulse (carotid) – place two finger tips in the indentation next to the Adam's apple.

Wrist pulse (radial) – place the tips of two or three fingers at the wrist on the thumb side.

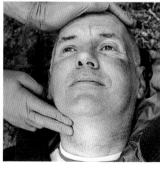
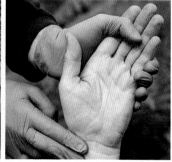

This is a skill you need to practise in order to become confident and competent; practise on yourself or your friends, until you can find pulses easily and quickly. Pulse rates vary enormously from one person to the next – the average resting adult rate ranges from about 60 to 100 beats per minute; but this can be as low as 50 to 70 for fit athletes or those on medication such as beta blockers. Child rates tend to be much higher depending on their age.

Photo: Claire Lynch

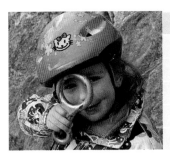

Age (years)	Beats per minute
less than 1	110 – 160
1 – 2	100 – 150
2 – 5	95 – 140
5 – 12	80 – 120
more than 12years	60 – 100

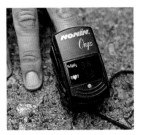

Fingertip pulse oximeter.

You may wish to consider carrying a fingertip pulse oximeter, which is a little device used to monitor a casualty's pulse and the amount of oxygen in their blood (oxygen saturation or SpO). A fit healthy adult normally has an oxygen saturation rate of between 95–99%, although this may vary with age, level of fitness, etc. These devices don't work very well on casualties with very cold hands or those wearing nail varnish, and can give error readings on casualties who are moving (such as shivering or experiencing a seizure) or casualties with dried blood on their fingers. However in the right circumstances a pulse oximeter can be a useful monitoring tool while you await rescue.

Skin colour

Skin colour is influenced by the blood circulating through the vessels and the skin pigment. In light-skinned people, a poor blood supply to the skin will cause the casualty to appear pale, white, ashen or grey. When there are low levels of oxygen in the blood, the skin, lips and nail beds can appear blue (cyanosis). With darker skin the changes may not be obvious, and a better assessment is to check the lining of the mouth and eyelids. The tissue should be flushed with blood. If very pale or white the circulation is poor.

Temperature

The only accurate way to take a core temperature outdoors is with a rectal thermometer. However, the general feeling is that although an accurate temperature reading is interesting, it is unlikely to change your treatment; therefore it is not recommended. The conscious casualty can usually say if they feel excessively hot or cold. Be aware however that in extreme cases of hypothermia (very cold) and hyperthermia (very hot) the casualty can complain of feeling too hot or too cold when in actual fact they are suffering from the opposite (see the chapter on **Heat and Cold Injuries and Conditions**).

4. Continue the activity or evacuate

1   **Scene survey**
Danger
What has happened?

2   **Initial assessment**
Level of response

Primary survey
Check **A**irway
Check **B**reathing
Check **C**irculation

Problem with the
Primary survey?
Dial 999/112

3   **Secondary survey**
Conscious casualty with injury
and/or medical condition

Take a history – S A M P L E
Injury?
Treat any injuries
Perform a head-to-toe if
appropriate
Medical conditions?
What's the problem?
Is there a past history of this
problem?
Are they, or you, carrying any
medication?
Take vital signs

4   **Continue the activity**   **Evacuate the casualty**

Self-evacuation

Dial 999/112
Request police – then
ask for mountain
rescue

After you have performed a **scene survey**, made your **initial assessment** including a **primary survey (ABC)**, performed a **secondary survey** and dealt with the injury and/or medical condition, you have to decide whether the casualty is able to **continue the activity** or needs to be **evacuated.**

Continue the activity

Before you can make this decision there are a whole host of questions you need to ask yourself, the casualty and if appropriate the rest of the group. Does the casualty want to continue? Do you agree with that decision? What effect has the injury or medical condition had on the rest of the group? Are they happy to continue? There are no hard and fast rules. If the decision is to continue, you (or a member of the casualty's group) will need to monitor the casualty carefully and re-assess the situation as the day progresses.

Evacuate: self-evacuation versus mountain rescue

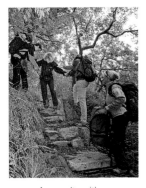

It may be possible for the casualty to walk themselves out of the remote setting, with a little help and support from others around. However, if the casualty has an injury to the legs this may be more of a challenge (see chapter on **Moving and Carrying a Casualty)**. Transporting a casualty can be an arduous task not only for those who offer their assistance but also the casualty themselves. The safety and welfare of all concerned are of vital importance – be realistic in your expectations and don't be afraid to re-assess the situation, and if necessary call for help.

If you decide to call for the rescue services, you should insulate the casualty from the ground and provide shelter. All information gathered during your **remote casualty assessment** should preferably be written on a **casualty report form** and handed to the rescue services when they arrive (see the chapter on **Working with Rescue Services)**.

A casualty with an injured ankle, being helped down a path.

Summary: dealing with a conscious casualty

1   **Scene survey**
Danger
What has happened?

2   **Initial assessment**
Level of response

Primary survey
Check **A**irway
Check **B**reathing
Check **C**irculation

Problem with the
Primary survey?
Dial 999/112

3   **Secondary survey**
Conscious casualty with injury
and/or medical condition

Take a history – S A M P L E
Injury?
Treat any injuries
Perform a head-to-toe if
appropriate
Medical conditions?
What's the problem?
Is there a past history of this
problem?
Are they, or you, carrying any
medication?
Take vital signs

4   **Continue the activity**   **Evacuate the casualty**

Self-evacuation

Dial 999/112
Request police – then
ask for mountain
rescue

OUTDOOR FIRST AID

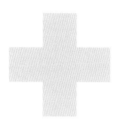

2. THE UNCONSCIOUS CASUALTY

There are many reasons why a casualty becomes unconscious, some medical, others through injury. In reality the reason why they are unconscious is not hugely important; your main concern is the fact they **are** unconscious. Before embarking on how to treat the unconscious casualty, it is suggested you familiarise yourself with how to deal with a conscious casualty (see previous chapter in which the **remote casualty assessment** is presented in detail).

The unconscious casualty

Being unconscious puts the casualty at risk on two levels. First (and critically), they lose the ability to keep their airway clear and open; second, they can no longer protect themselves from the environment. On occasions, unfortunately, the unconscious casualty may stop breathing; it is important therefore that you are trained appropriately to deal with this situation and are aware of the issues surrounding resuscitation in a remote setting.

Remote casualty assessment: unconscious

The assessment for an unconscious casualty is more detailed than that of a conscious casualty, particularly in the **primary survey**: the airway and breathing will need to be checked thoroughly and frequently. Any casualty who remains unconscious for whatever reason will need to be evacuated to hospital as a matter of urgency.

The assessment is divided into three levels, which will be explained in more detail later.

1. Scene survey.

2. Initial assessment including the primary survey.

3a. Unconscious breathing OR **3b.** Unconscious NOT breathing.

1 **Scene survey**
Danger

2 **Initial assessment**
Level of response

Primary survey
Check **A**irway
Check **B**reathing

3a

Unconscious breathing

Check **C**irculation

Unconscious
Dial 999/112
Request police – then ask for
mountain rescue

Secondary survey
Unconscious casualty

Safe airway position

Monitor vital signs
until help arrives

3b

Unconscious NOT breathing

Dial 999/112
Request police – then ask for
mountain rescue
Available *AED?

If appropriate start basic life
support – CPR

*Automated External Defibrillator

1. Scene survey

The **scene survey** involves rapidly assessing any actual or potential dangers to yourself, the casualty (and others), and forming some initial impressions about what has happened.

The scene survey is discussed in detail in the previous chapter **Dealing with a conscious casualty.** What is important to re-emphasise here is that you must only approach a scene if it is safe for you to do so.

1

Scene survey
Danger
What has happened?

Initial assessment
Level of response

Primary survey
Check **A**irway
Check **B**reathing

Unconscious breathing

Unconscious NOT breathing

Check **C**irculation

Dial 999/112
Request police – then ask for
mountain rescue
Available AED?

Unconscious
Dial 999/112
Request police – then ask for
mountain rescue

If appropriate start Basic Life
Support – CPR

Secondary survey
Unconscious casualty

Safe airway position

Monitor vital signs
until help arrives

2. Initial assessment – primary survey

After the **scene survey,** move on to the **initial assessment**. Establish the casualty's **level of response** (are they conscious or unconscious), and if appropriate, shout for help from other bystanders. Start your **primary survey,** with checks to the **A**irway and establish if they are **B**reathing.

Scene survey
Danger

2   **Initial assessment**
Level of response
Shout for HELP!

Primary survey
Check **A**irway
Check **B**reathing

Unconscious breathing

Check **C**irculation

Unconscious
Dial 999/112
Request police – then ask for
mountain rescue

Secondary survey
Unconscious casualty

Safe airway position

Monitor vital signs
until help arrives

Unconscious **NOT** breathing

Dial 999/112
Request police – then ask for
mountain rescue
Available AED?

If appropriate start basic life
support – CPR

Level of response: conscious or unconscious? (AVPU)

Assess their level of response using the **AVPU** scale (**A**lert, **V**oice, **P**ain, or **U**nresponsive). If the casualty is not **A**lert (and conscious), try squeezing their shoulders gently and use your **V**oice to ask them a question, such as "Can you hear me?" or "Can you tell me what happened?"; speak loudly and clearly. If they do not respond to your voice apply a **P**ain stimulus (usually a pinch just above the ear lobe). If they do not respond to **V**oice or **P**ain they are said to be **U**nresponsive.

AVPU SCALE OF RESPONSIVENESS

Conscious

A = Alert

The conscious casualty is Alert, speaks clearly and responds to questions. They spontaneously open their eyes when you approach, react to your voice (though they may be confused) and appear to be aware of, and react to, their environment.

Unconscious

V = Verbal stimulus

The casualty makes some kind of response when you speak to them (it may be necessary for you to raise your voice or even shout). The casualty may open their eyes, or the response may be as subtle as a quiet grunt or moan, or perhaps slight movement of a limb when prompted by the first aider.

P = Pain stimulus

If the casualty does not respond to your voice then apply some form of pain stimulus. When a painful stimulus is applied the casualty may react in some way; move, groan or stir.

U = Unresponsive

The casualty does not respond to any stimulus.

The casualty is given the best level of response that they are able to **maintain**. For example if when you arrive the casualty is unresponsive, but over the last hour they have been responding to your **V**oice they are said to be 'unconscious but responding to voice'. It is important, however, that you record the initial response and all subsequent changes.

If you find yourself alone with an unconscious casualty, it would be sensible to shout for help.

The primary survey – ABCs

As with the conscious casualty, the primary survey – **A**irway, **B**reathing, and **C**irculation – is part of your rapid initial assessment and guides you towards detecting any life-threatening conditions that need your immediate attention.

Check airway

The unconscious casualty's airway is particularly at risk from the tongue falling back and blocking the back of the throat, thus stopping air from entering the lungs. If the tongue partially blocks the airway, you may hear snoring or gurgling noises. Snoring unconscious casualties are not asleep; they have a blocked airway which needs sorting out urgently! Any objects or fluid in the mouth such as food, broken teeth, vomit or blood must be removed or cleared.

Clearing the airway

Remove any obvious foreign objects (such as sweets, chewing gum etc.) from the mouth with your fingers; do not randomly stick your finger in their mouth and wildly fish around. Vomit and blood pose a different challenge, either you drain the liquid, or they drown in it! The easiest and safest way of doing this is to place them into a safe airway position (sometimes also known as the recovery position), ensuring the mouth is lower than the back of the throat, allowing any fluid to drain away. With the injured casualty, also consider the possibility of a spinal injury and if possible use a **modified** safe airway position (see chapter on **Spine and back injuries**). However it is important to stress that a clear and open airway always has priority over a possible spinal injury.

Opening an airway

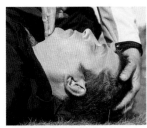

Open the airway using a simple head tilt, chin lift manoeuvre; this brings the tongue off the back of the throat. If you suspect a spinal injury and there are two of you, use the alternative jaw thrust technique which avoids unnecessary movement of the neck. The person who performs the jaw thrust must stay in that position to keep the airway open.

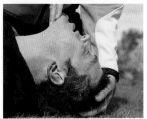

HEAD TILT, CHIN LIFT

Place your hand on the casualty's forehead and the fingertips of the other hand on the bone part of the chin.

Gently tilt the head back while lifting the chin upwards.

JAW THRUST

Place your finger tips at the corner of the jaw bone by the ear lobe.

Gently push the lower jaw up towards the sky, taking care not to move the head.

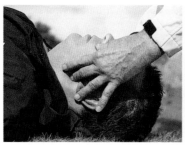 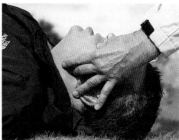

Check breathing

Once the airway has been assessed and opened, check for **normal** breathing. Look down the line of the chest to see if it rises and falls. Place your cheek above their mouth and nose to listen and feel for the sounds and signs of breathing.

To check breathing, if necessary open the jacket or other clothing and place your hand directly onto the chest.

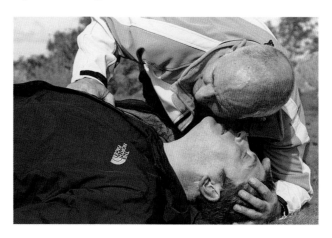

Take no more than ten seconds to complete this, by which time you need to establish if the casualty is breathing normally or not. The irregular gasping noise you sometimes hear when a casualty's heart has stopped (agonal gasps) is not 'normal' and is treated as if the casualty is not breathing.

If the casualty is breathing normally you can move on to your circulation checks.

3a. Unconscious casualty breathing

When your **scene survey** and **initial assessment** are complete, and you have started your **primary survey** establishing the casualty has an **A**irway and is **B**reathing, move on to check for **C**irculation. You also need to **summon help**, perform a **secondary survey**, ensure your casualty is in a safe airway position and then **monitor vital signs** until help arrives.

Scene survey
Danger

Initial assessment
Level of response

Primary survey
Check **A**irway
Check **B**reathing

3a

Unconscious breathing	Unconscious NOT breathing
Check **C**irculation	Dial 999/112 Request police – then ask for mountain rescue Available AED?
Unconscious Dial 999/112 Request police – then ask for mountain rescue	If appropriate start basic life support – CPR
Secondary survey Unconscious casualty	
Safe airway position	
Monitor vital signs until help arrives	

Check circulation

The priority here is to identify external catastrophic life-threatening bleeding and urgently stop it. Checks also need to be made to identify other potential areas of life-threatening internal bleeding, such as into the chest cavity, abdomen, broken pelvis and/or thigh bones. Assess the casualty's skin colour – are they turning very pale, or blue? – and if possible take a pulse. A pulse rate of over 100 beats per minute may indicate the casualty is going into blood loss shock, which is an emergency and must also be treated (see chapter on **Life-threatening Bleeding and Shock**).

If the casualty remains unconscious summon help. Dial 999/112, request **police**, then ask for **mountain rescue**. If possible ask someone else to do this for you and continue onto your secondary survey.

Secondary survey – unconscious casualty

Start your **head-to-toe examination;** this is identical to that performed on the conscious casualty (see previous chapter on **Dealing with a Conscious Casualty**). The unconscious casualty is unable to tell you if they feel pain therefore be thorough in your assessment checking the whole body, comparing one side to the other. You will also need to remove any bulky objects from the pockets, such as mobile phones or keys, and check if the casualty is wearing any medical alerts.

Medical alerts

Some individuals who have a medical condition may carry or wear a medical alert; usually a piece of jewellery. These 'alerts' typically include details of a condition the wearer wishes to make known, such as allergies to certain things, or a medical condition. Not everyone who has a condition wears a medical alert, and not all medical alerts look the same, but they can be a useful indicator of a known medical condition.

Check the casualty's wrist and neck for a medical alert worn as a necklace, bracelet or watch. Read the information on the disk and pass the details onto the rescue services.

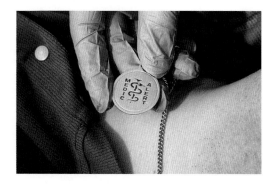

Safe airway position

The unconscious casualty's airway is at risk from two things; first the tongue falling back and obstructing the passage of air, stopping the casualty breathing, and second the possibility of fluid such as vomit quietly working its way to the back of the throat and the casualty breathing it into the lungs. For this reason, the casualty is best managed in a safe airway position, which is any position where the mouth is lower than the back of the throat so that the tongue is forward and any fluid can drain away.

SAFE AIRWAY POSITION

How to place a casualty with a suspected spinal injury into a safe airway position is covered in the chapter on **Spine and Back Injuries**.

Remove the casualty's glasses, if present. Kneel by the casualty's side. If they are on a slope do this from the down-hill side. Straighten the legs out if possible. Take the casualty's arm nearest you and place it out to the side, with the palm upwards.

Take the casualty's other hand and interlock your thumb with their thumb leaving your fingers free.

Bring this arm across their chest and place the casualty's hand (interlocked with yours) next to their cheek on your side of the casualty. With your other hand take the knee on the far side and bend it, sliding the foot up towards the casualty's bottom.

Keeping one hand against the cheek, pull on the knee rotating the casualty towards you. Concentrate on controlling and protecting the head during the move – failure to do this could result in the head hitting the ground. Stabilise the casualty by bending the leg you have brought over to make a right angle.   ...

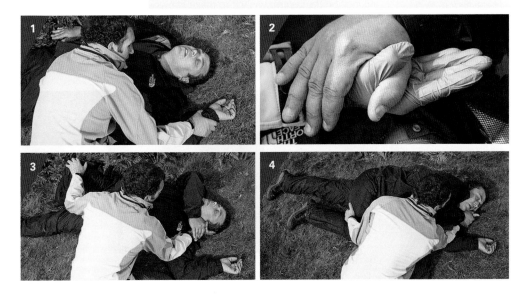

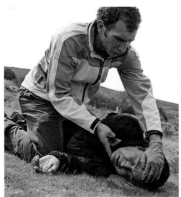
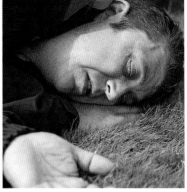

Remove your hand from the cheek, re-position the head and open the airway with a chin lift, head tilt. The mouth should be lower than the back of the throat so that the tongue sits forward and any fluid can drain away.

As a general rule, if a casualty has been left in a safe airway position for 30 minutes, the advice is to roll them onto their back and then roll them onto their other side in order to avoid pressure sores. In the remote setting this may be difficult due to their location, or the type and number of injuries they have sustained.

Monitor vital signs

If possible, insulate the casualty from the ground, provide shelter then monitor their vital signs until help arrives. Taking and monitoring vital signs (covered in the chapter on **Dealing with a Conscious Casualty**) can help identify any problems and may also indicate changes in the casualty's condition. These can be taken initially during the secondary survey and then monitored while you await the arrival of the rescue services. Your findings should be written down on a **casualty report form** or a note pad.

LOOK OUT FOR

Level of response – AVPU.

Breathing.

Pulse.

Skin colour.

Temperature.

3b. Unconscious casualty NOT breathing

When your **scene survey** and **initial assessment** are complete, and you have started your **primary survey** establishing the casualty has a clear and open **A**irway but is **NOT B**reathing, you must now stop and immediately **summon help**, request any **available AED** then if appropriate start basic life support (CPR).

Scene survey
Danger

Initial assessment
Level of response

Primary survey
Check **A**irway
Check **B**reathing

3b

Unconscious NOT breathing

Unconscious breathing

Check **C**irculation

Dial 999/112 Request police – then ask for mountain rescue Available AED?

Unconscious
Dial 999/112
Request police – then ask for mountain rescue

If appropriate start basic life support – CPR

Secondary survey
Unconscious casualty

Adult 30 chest compressions 2 breaths 30 chest compressions 2 breaths Continue …

Safe airway position

Monitor vital signs
until help arrives

Dial 999/112 – summon mountain rescue – available AED?

A casualty who is not breathing has a primary survey problem, therefore you need to urgently dial 999/112, request **police**, and then ask for **mountain rescue**. If possible ask someone to do this for you so that you can continue with your assessment and, if appropriate, treatment.

You should also consider whether an Automated External Defibrillator (AED) is available and reasonably close. An AED is a little machine which when attached by 'pads' to the casualty's chest can deliver an electric shock that may, in certain circumstances, restore a normal heart rhythm.

In the remote setting you are unlikely to have immediate access to an AED. Having said that, there is one in the summit café of Snowdon, the highest mountain in England and Wales, which is accessible during the café's opening times between the end of March and late October. It is also not unheard of for walking groups of a more mature nature to actually carry their own!

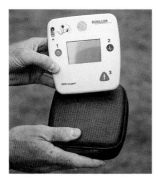

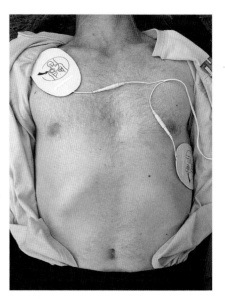

This Automated External Defibrillator (AED) is pocket sized, weighs 490g and about the length of a pen.

Look at the drawing on the back of the pads for the correct positioning. One pad is placed below the casualty's right collar bone above the nipple. The other pad is placed sideways over the ribs in line with the arm pit, below the left breast. Once the pads are in place plug the pads connector firmly into the AED unit.

Chain of survival

For a casualty who is not breathing the best chance they have is for you to rapidly dial 999/112, give early cardiopulmonary resuscitation (CPR), defibrillate quickly using an AED and then get the casualty to hospital and advanced care as fast as possible, This is known as the **chain of survival.**

Early help	Early CPR	Early defibrillator	Early transfer
Dial 999/112 immediately, request **police**, then ask for **mountain rescue**. Is there an Automated External Defibrillator (AED) available close-by?	**To buy time,** Once you know help is being sought and any available AED has been requested you can start chest compressions and breathing for the casualty.	**To restart the heart** the casualty urgently needs an AED to deliver a controlled shock to try and kick start the heart into a normal rhythm.	**Transfer to hospital.** The casualty needs to be immediately evacuated to hospital.

Urgent evacuation to hospital.

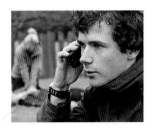

This chain of survival relies on the **early** delivery of each of the actions. Unfortunately this concept does not really suit the remote situation, when help can be some hours away and an AED simply not to hand. However there always exists the possibility of a helicopter already airborne and near to your location, with an AED and trained paramedic on board who may be able to give rapid and very specialised treatment.

If appropriate start basic life support (CPR)

If a casualty is **not** breathing, this is an indicator to start basic life support (BLS). BLS involves supporting circulation by performing chest compressions and breathing for the casualty – together these are known as cardiopulmonary resuscitation (CPR).

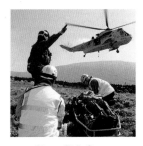

When the heart stops, blood is no longer pumped around the body to the vital organs. These become starved of oxygen and if this is not restored, the vital organs will die. By compressing the chest and the underlying heart, the first aider can help push the blood out of the heart and around the body. To help maintain the oxygen level in the blood, the first aider may also breathe for the casualty.

Photo: Elidir Owen

How to do CPR

The current sequence for adult CPR is to start with 30 chest compressions, followed by two breaths and then repeat (this is also suitable for children with the modification that the chest should be compressed by one third of its depth and that the compressions should be performed with one hand only). Should you feel unable or unwilling to perform rescue breathing then the guidance is for you to perform chest compressions only.

If you wish to become competent at performing CPR you will need to attend a suitable first aid course. For the most up-to-date information on resuscitation visit www.resus.org.uk

CHEST COMPRESSIONS

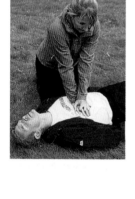

Kneel by the side of the casualty, roughly level with their chest, and place the heel of one hand in the **centre** of the casualty's chest (the lower half of the breast bone). There is no need to remove clothing, unless they are wearing significantly bulky layers such as duvet jackets.

Place your other hand on top of the first and interlock your fingers. Pull the fingers back and clear of the chest. Only the heel of the hand should make contact with the chest to avoid pushing onto the ribs.

With straight arms, lean directly over the casualty's chest and push down vertically about 5–6cm.

After each compression, release the pressure without losing contact between your hands and the casualty's chest. Compress the chest 30 times aiming for a rate of between 100-120 compressions per minute.

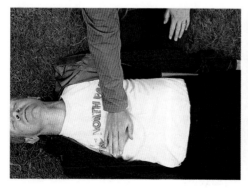

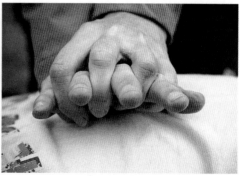

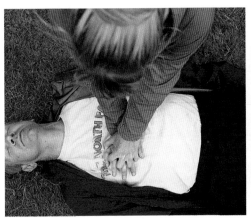
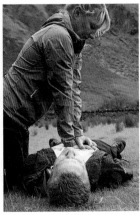
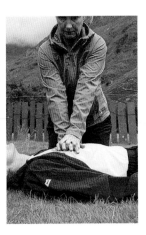

BREATHING FOR THE CASUALTY

Open the airway (head tilt chin lift), pinch the soft part of the casualty's nose. Allow the mouth to open while maintaining the chin lift.

Take a normal breath in and place your lips around the casualty's mouth creating a complete seal. Blow slowly and steadily into the mouth (**while** watching their chest rise) to mimic normal breathing.

Maintain the head tilt, chin lift. Take your mouth away from the casualty and watch the chest fall as they breathe out. You take a fresh breath in, and then blow into the casualty once more. The two breaths should take no more than five seconds in total.

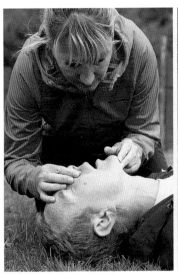
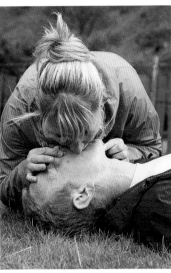
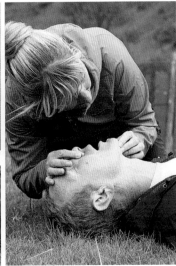

Face shields and pocket masks

These are produced to provide protection from infection (for both the casualty and the first aider) while performing rescue breathing. They provide a barrier preventing direct contact between the casualty's mouth and the first aider.

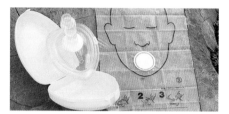

Face shield and pocket mask. Photo: Brian Wills

When to start, continue or stop CPR

Urban first aid courses guide you towards **always** starting CPR and once started not to stop until the emergency services arrive, another first aider takes over, the casualty shows signs of regaining consciousness – such as coughing, opening eyes, speaking or moving purposefully **and** breathing normally – or you become so exhausted you can no longer continue. This approach does not conveniently fit into the more remote setting and I raised this issue with the UK resuscitation council; their reply is below.

"The Resuscitation Council (UK) recognises that skill acquisition and retention in resuscitation training is a problem, particularly for lay people. Where possible, therefore, the basic life support guidelines have been simplified to aid learning, and are designed to apply to the majority of situations when CPR will be needed. We deliberately do not issue detailed guidelines on resuscitation in situations such as mountaineering, but recommend that guidance should be based on the general principles of CPR, modified by those aware of the unique circumstances".

Sarah Mitchell
Resuscitation Council (UK)

Some would argue that teaching CPR on a first aid course geared towards the remote setting is a complete waste of time as the casualty stands virtually no chance of surviving. Others would argue that if each stage of the **chain of survival** can be quickly applied, then there is no reason why a life could not be saved. Unfortunately every year people in remote settings throughout the UK are faced with the dilemma of dealing with a casualty who has stopped breathing; it is, therefore, worth considering some of the issues surrounding CPR in this unique environment.

Starting CPR

If a casualty is not breathing, the guidance is for you to dial 999/112, request any available AED and then start CPR. In the remote setting, however, there are some exceptions to this rule, based on many years of research and experience from American Search and Rescue organisations.

When CPR is considered futile

The decision to start CPR in the remote setting remains with the first aider and nobody else, but there are a number of situations in which research has indicated resuscitation may actually be ineffective. These include the following.

- When the heart has stopped due to some massive injury; this can include a severe head or chest injury.

- The person appears dead: from lethal injuries (such as decapitation) or the presence of rigor mortis (stiffness in death).

- A drowned casualty who has been underwater for more than 90 minutes.

- The casualty is frozen solid and the chest is not compressible.

When to give prolonged CPR

- The drowned casualty: when they have been under the water for less than 30 minutes.

- Avalanche casualty: unless the airway is packed with snow.

- After the heart has stopped from a lightning strike.

When to stop CPR

Once you have started CPR there are occasions when it is indicated you should/may stop.

- The casualty recovers: the casualty shows signs of regaining consciousness, such as coughing, opening their eyes, speaking or moving purposefully **and** breathing normally.

- You become too exhausted to continue.

- The situation becomes unsafe for you to continue.

- The casualty is declared dead by a doctor (it is important to check this is a doctor of medicine and that they are appropriately qualified to declare death).

- A member of the rescue services arrives and ask you to stop.

  When faced with the dilemma of a casualty who is no longer breathing there will be a number of other factors that influence your CPR decision making. For instance, the casualty is a friend or relative, the next of kin is begging you to do something, you come across a situation but have responsibilities as a party leader to care for others. The guidance offered in this chapter attempts to help you to make an informed choice as to when to start, when to aggressively continue and when to consider stopping CPR in the remote setting.

Summary: the unconscious casualty

1

Scene survey
Danger
What has happened?

2

Initial assessment
Level of response
Shout for HELP!

Primary survey
Check **A**irway
Check **B**reathing

3a

Unconscious breathing

Check **C**irculation

Unconscious
Dial 999/112
Request police – then ask for
mountain rescue

Secondary survey
Unconscious casualty

Safe airway position

Monitor vital signs
until help arrives

3b

Unconscious NOT breathing

Dial 999/112
Request police – then ask for
mountain rescue
Available *AED?

If appropriate start basic life
support – CPR

Adult
30 chest compressions
2 breaths
30 chest compressions
2 breaths

Continue …

*Automated External Defibrillator

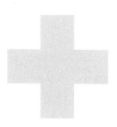

3. BREATHING PROBLEMS

Shortness of breath with exercise is a common complaint. In the remote setting your challenge will be to work out if you can manage the problem yourself, or whether this is an emergency that requires urgent evacuation.

Breathing

When we breathe, air is drawn in through the mouth and nose, and then travels down the tubes (air passages) of the throat, voice box and windpipe. The tubes then branch into two, sending air into the left and right lung. Inside the lungs, air passages continue to branch into ever decreasing tubes and end in little sacs (alveoli). It is within these alveoli that the lung transfers oxygen into the blood stream and removes carbon dioxide.

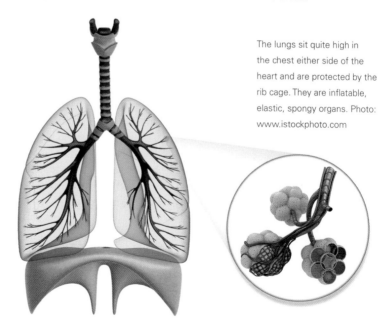

The lungs sit quite high in the chest either side of the heart and are protected by the rib cage. They are inflatable, elastic, spongy organs. Photo: www.istockphoto.com

How we breathe

Breathing involves two actions; inhaling (the in phase), then exhaling (the out phase), followed by a pause. The brain monitors levels of carbon dioxide and oxygen in the blood. When carbon dioxide levels become too high and oxygen becomes too low, a message is sent to the muscles between the ribs and the large muscle sitting underneath the lungs (diaphragm), telling them to contract. It is a combination of all these things working together that enables us to breathe.

BREATHING IN

The diaphragm muscle (at the bottom of the lungs) moves down, while the ribs move up and outwards. This produces a negative pressure and air is drawn in.

BREATHING OUT

Muscles between the ribs and the diaphragm relax; the ribs move back down and in. The lungs recoil back to their original position and air flows out.

Normal breathing

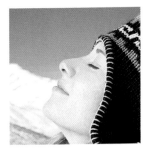

Photo:
www.istockphoto.com

Normal breathing appears effortless. There is a smooth flow of air moving in and out of the lungs, seen as a regular rise and fall movement on both sides of the chest. The conscious casualty who is breathing normally is able to speak clearly using unhurried sentences. Be vigilant, however, for breathing that is either excessively deep or shallow, as well as extremely fast or very slow. It would be a cause for concern if an adult casualty was breathing at a rate of less than 10 or more than 30 breaths per minute. In essence, it should mimic your own normal breathing.

A casualty who is struggling to breathe may appear to be working hard, sometimes using other muscles around the neck and upper chest. They often sit forward using their hands to grasp something, with their chin and head thrust slightly forwards. The conscious casualty having difficulty breathing would use clipped half sentences, single words or even grunts. Their skin would also appear pale or blue (cyanotic).

Agonal gasps

This is a strange intermittent gasping noise that sometimes happens after a cardiac arrest, and can be mistaken for breathing. Eye witnesses describe this as a "weird noise" which is "really slow and infrequent" and sounds like "choking or gurgling". These gasps are not effective breathing and their presence should be an indicator to start cardiopulmonary resuscitation (CPR).

Breathing problems and emergencies

This chapter deals with breathing related problems and emergencies. You may be able to manage some of these yourself such as choking, hyperventilation or a minor chest injury; others, like airway burns and a severe allergic reaction (anaphylaxis), will require urgent removal to hospital.

Choking

Choking refers to a blockage of the upper airway – either partial or complete – which stops an individual from breathing effectively. Choking is an emergency and a few simple prompt actions by you can make a huge difference.

Mild choking

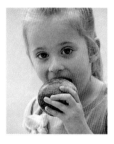

Adults and children tend to choke while eating. Children can also choke while playing.

During mild choking the airway is only partially blocked and the individual is usually able to speak, cry, cough and importantly, breathe. Typically the casualty is able to clear the blockage themselves.

LOOK OUT FOR	
Adult	**Child**
Coughing, gagging, and wheezing.	Crying or speaks when questioned.
Panic, sometimes pointing to the throat.	A loud cough.
	Able to take a breath before coughing.
Able to speak.	
	Alert.

WHAT TO DO

Ask the question 'are you choking?' if yes, ask them to 'cough!'

Effective coughing:

Continue to encourage them to cough – do nothing else.

Remove any obvious obstruction from the mouth.

Continue to monitor in case the airway becomes fully blocked or the choking becomes severe.

Severe choking

When choking is severe the casualty will not be able to speak, cry, cough or breathe. Without your assistance they will eventually become unconscious and possibly die.

LOOK OUT FOR

Complete obstruction:

Both hands clutch at the throat.

Unable to cough (in children a quiet or silent cough).

Unable to speak or breathe.

Skin of the face and lips turn blue (cyanosed).

May become unconscious.

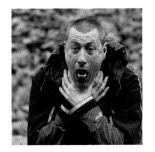
Photo: Brian Wills

WHAT TO DO

Initially ask the question 'are you choking?' encourage them to 'cough!' If they are unable to cough:

Stand to the side and slightly behind the casualty and lean them forwards; support the chest with one of your hands.

Give up to five sharp blows between the shoulder blades with the heel of the hand, checking to see if the object has cleared after each blow (children: if possible position the child head down or if small enough across the lap). ...

If back blows fail, give up to five abdominal thrusts. Stand behind the casualty; wrap your arms around their rib cage. Lean the casualty forwards, clench your fist and place it between their belly button and the bottom of the breast bone. Hold your fist firmly with your other hand and pull sharply in and upwards.

Repeat back blows and abdominal thrusts until the airway is clear.

If you are unable to clear the airway, or they become unconscious:

Dial 999/112 – request police – then ask for mountain rescue.

If they become unconscious follow your **ABC**s. If they are not breathing start basic life support (CPR).

Drowning

Drowning refers to a casualty who has been under the surface of the water (or a liquid) and experiences breathing impairment. Your casualty's condition may vary from conscious and cold but feeling okay – though at potential risk of breathing complications later – through to the unconscious cardiac arrest.

Your safety comes first! It is vital you assess your own safety as a priority. Too many well meaning people die every year while trying to assist someone drowning, or rescuing their pet.
Photo:
www.istockphoto.com

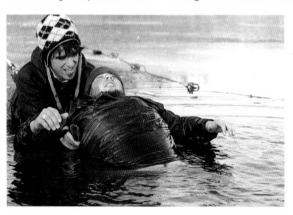

During land based activities there have, unfortunately, been instances of people being swept away and drowned while attempting to cross fast flowing rivers or streams. Many footpaths can be found near water such as approach paths to certain climbs, or tourist paths alongside rivers and waterfalls. A slip, trip, or fall could result in some kind of injury and end with the casualty in water.

As the casualty enters the water there is an initial panic and gasp, a period of breath holding, followed by rapid uncontrollable breathing. The casualty will be fully clothed, restricting movement in the water, making staying on the surface difficult. As they disappear under water the eventual lack of oxygen and not being able to get rid of the carbon dioxide, compounded by exhaustion, will cause the casualty to become unconscious, stop breathing (respiratory arrest) and eventually go into cardiac arrest.

WHAT TO DO

Remove the casualty from the water – do not put yourself in danger.

Conscious

If conscious look for signs of water in the lungs such as:

- Chest pain.

- Coughing.

- Breathing difficulties.

- White or pink foam around the nostrils or mouth.

Insulate from the ground and provide shelter, this casualty is at risk of hypothermia.

Evacuate the casualty and take to hospital for further assessment.

Unconscious

Dial 999/112 – request police – then ask for mountain rescue.

Follow your **ABC**s – if not breathing start basic life support (CPR).

Complications

Casualties who have been rescued after being submerged in water can go on to develop a life-threatening breathing problem up to 72 hours after the incident. It is therefore recommended that anyone who has been under the water (even intermittently) and is thought to have breathed in water must be seen in hospital.

Chest injuries

The chest extends from the lower part of the neck to the diaphragm (upper abdomen). It is encased in the front by the breast and collar bones, at the back by the spine and shoulder blades, and is encircled by the ribs. The upper and main part of the rib cage surrounds the lungs and the heart, while the lower ribs protect organs such as the liver, spleen, and stomach.

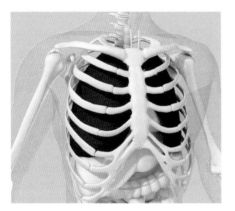

The human chest.
Photo: www.istockphoto.com

Injuries to the chest are either open or closed. Closed chest injuries do not break through the skin and are generally caused by some form of blunt trauma which can break ribs, collapse and bruise lungs, injure the heart and damage some big blood vessels. Open chest injuries on the other hand involve something penetrating the chest wall itself; either from an external source, for instance from an ice axe, or internally, for example being pierced by a broken rib.

Broken ribs

Most rib fractures are not usually serious; however the discomfort and pain can be quite intense and make breathing difficult. Treatment is limited to offering pain relief and evacuating the casualty from the remote environment. Be cautious when you suspect broken lower ribs, they can puncture internal organs, such as the liver or spleen: monitor for signs of shock and, if concerned, arrange for urgent evacuation.

A casualty may break one or more ribs and, on occasions, break the same rib in more than one place (flail chest). A flail chest is quite difficult to see initially (unless it's particularly large), as the chest muscles go into spasm and tend to keep everything in place. The casualty will be working extremely hard to breathe and eventually become exhausted; as this happens the flail will become more noticeable. When the casualty breathes in, the rib cage moves up and out; the flail segment will move in and vice versa.

The treatment is to pad over the segment enabling it to move in time with the rest of the chest. Ask the casualty to breathe in, then using a bulky pad, place it over the damaged area and secure in place with tape. An alternative method is to simply ask the casualty to support the area with their own hand which helps to reduce pain and aid breathing. Flail chest fractures have the potential to be serious if the lung underneath is damaged. Monitor this casualty carefully for signs of deterioration and if necessary evacuate urgently.

Collapsed lung

A lung can collapse spontaneously without warning (very tall thin people are prone to this), or after a blunt trauma or a penetrating injury. Damage to the lining of the chest can cause air to escape into the gap between the chest wall and lung. This breaks the 'seal', causing the lung to detach and collapse.

Collapsed lung – blunt injury

The severity of the symptoms from a collapsed lung (closed pneumothorax) will depend on how much air gets into the space between the chest wall lining and the lung itself. For some only a small segment collapses, for others it may be the whole lung.

On rare occasions the lung surface itself will tear, creating a hole which allows air to pass into the chest cavity, but will not allow it back out. With every breath the tension within the enclosed chest cavity increases, squashing the other lung and the heart, stopping them from working properly. This is a serious medical emergency (tension pneumothorax) and without rapid medical attention will lead to death.

LOOK OUT FOR

History of an injury to the chest.

Shortness of breath.

Pain in the chest worse on breathing in.

In serious cases (tension pneumothorax):

Casualty complains 'I can't breathe'.

Very fast breathing.

Pale and clammy.

Symptoms continue to worsen.

WHAT TO DO

Sit the casualty down.

Examine the casualty. If breathing is not too difficult it may be possible for the casualty to walk unassisted.

This casualty benefits from painkillers.

If serious:

Dial 999/112 – request police – then ask for mountain rescue.

Insulate from the ground, provide shelter and monitor vital signs; level of response (AVPU), breathing and pulse.

If the casualty becomes unconscious place in a safe airway position. Roll them onto the injured side to enable the healthy lung to work effectively and monitor carefully.

Collapsed lung – penetrating injury

An open chest wound (open pneumothorax) large enough to allow air to enter from the outside (two thirds the diameter of the windpipe) can cause the lung to collapse. As air flows out of the chest cavity through the wound you may see bubbles of air and hear a noise – but often there is no sound at all.

LOOK OUT FOR

History of an injury to the chest.

On examination an obvious penetrating wound.

Difficulty breathing.

Chest pain.

WHAT TO DO

Dial 999/112 – request police – then ask for mountain rescue.

Sit the casualty down.

Examine the casualty and identify a penetrating chest wound.   ...

Seal the wound **immediately** using an airtight dressing.

Improvise using the cellophane packaging from a wound dressing and tape into place around two sides and top. The bottom is left free, creating a one-way valve that stops air from entering the chest cavity but allows it to escape. Monitor this casualty carefully for any signs of deterioration after dressing. If breathing and chest pain become severe or rapidly worsen, remove your dressing immediately! This could be contributing to a more dangerous chest condition developing (tension pneumothorax).

Insulate from the ground, provide shelter and monitor vital signs; level of response (AVPU), breathing and pulse.

If the casualty becomes unconscious place in a safe airway position. Roll them onto the injured side to allow the healthy lung to work effectively and monitor carefully.

Bleeding into the chest cavity

On occasions the injury may cause bleeding into the space between the chest wall lining and the lung (haemothorax), causing the lung to collapse. The chest cavity can expand to hold a significant amount of blood, sufficient to cause the casualty to go into shock. At a basic first aid level, this injury can be difficult to detect; it may be that your ability to identify a casualty with breathing difficulties and signs and symptoms of shock alerts you.

Inhalation injuries

Inhalation injuries may be due to being either trapped in a fire or exposure to poisonous gases in an enclosed space. In the remote setting the poisonous gas is likely to be carbon monoxide from poor ventilation in a confined shelter while cooking, or near an open fire.

Airway burns and smoke inhalation

Any burn to the face from fire should alert you to the possibility of both an airway and a smoke inhalation injury. Smoke is a bigger killer than fire itself. Not only is it low in oxygen but it can also contain poisonous fumes from the material being burned. Damage to the lungs and airways may not be quite as obvious as burns to the skin and can take many hours to develop.

If airway burns are suspected it is vital that you pass the emergency services a detailed history of exactly what happened; the casualty may not be able to do this themselves. Photo: www.istockphoto.com

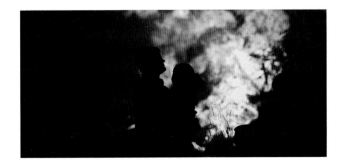

Take a thorough history of what happened, including: the length of time the casualty was in the confined space (particularly if the casualty was asleep), the substances that were burning, and whether the casualty already has a pre-existing medical condition which causes breathing difficulties, such as asthma.

LOOK OUT FOR

Any of the following:

Unconscious.

Signs of soot around the mouth and nose.

Difficulty breathing.

Specifically:

Airway Burn	**Smoke Inhalation**
Evidence of burns to the face and mouth.	Rapid noisy breathing.
Coughing with soot coloured spit.	Coughing and wheezing.
Swollen tongue.	Burning sensation in the nose and mouth
Singed nasal hair, eyelashes or eye brows.	Wheezing, gasping or breathlessness.
Sore throat, hoarseness or croakiness.	

WHAT TO DO

Assess for **danger** before you attempt to remove a casualty from a fire, or fume-filled environment.

If the incident involves a blast and the casualty has been thrown a distance, consider a possible spinal injury and treat accordingly.

Sit the casualty down in the fresh air and start your **ABC**s.

Assess how well the casualty is breathing.

If there is evidence of an airway burn or smoke inhalation:

Dial 999/112 – request police – then ask for mountain rescue.

Examine the casualty for any other injuries.

Insulate from the ground, provide shelter and monitor vital signs; level of response (AVPU), breathing and pulse.

If they become unconscious place into a safe airway position and monitor until help arrives. If breathing stops be prepared to start basic life support (CPR).

Carbon monoxide poisoning

Carbon monoxide is colourless, odourless and tasteless. It doesn't irritate so is actually very difficult to detect. In the remote setting carbon monoxide poisoning can happen in mountain bothies, small tents and particularly snow holes; in fact any enclosed area where you are cooking, using candles or there is an open fire. The symptoms are pretty vague and can be mistaken for other conditions, like tiredness, flu and even food poisoning.

LOOK OUT FOR

Symptons of **mild carbon monoxide poisoning** may include:

Headache.

Tiredness.

Abdominal pain, nausea and vomiting.

Muscle weakness – general flu-like symptoms.   ...

Symptons of **severe carbon monoxide poisoning** may include:

Rapid difficult breathing.

Irregular heart rate.

Confusion.

Dilated pupils.

Unconsciousness.

WHAT TO DO

Move the casualty into the fresh air, then:

If conscious

Sit the casualty down.

If symptoms improve, identify the source of the carbon monoxide poisoning (this is usually poor or inadequate ventilation in the shelter) and rectify.

If you are unsure if the risk still exists do **not** return to the shelter.

If you do return to the shelter, continue to monitor for signs and symptoms of carbon monoxide poisoning. Do not go to sleep if there is any doubt that you have sorted out the problem.

If unconscious

Dial 999/112 – request police – then ask for mountain rescue.

Place the casually in a safe airway position.

Insulate from the ground, provide shelter and monitor vital signs; level of response (AVPU), breathing and pulse.

If breathing stops be prepared to start basic life support (CPR).

Photo:
www.istockphoto.com

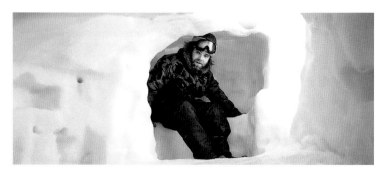

Be aware of the symptoms of carbon monoxide – particularly a headache and nausea – and take regular trips outside to see if the symptoms go away.

DANGER

Cooking: tents and snow holes

Keep your stove highly pressurised, avoid low flames and prolonged simmering. Use small pans.

Inadequate ventilation: tents

Keep the outlet for carbon monoxide as high as possible and the fresh air vent as low as possible.

Inadequate ventilation: snow holes

Make sure you punch a ventilation hole (or holes) in the roof, and never completely block off the door.

Tent: icing and snow cover

Clear ice and snow from the tent regularly to keep the fabric breathable.

Asthma

Asthma involves the constriction of the airways inside the lungs. A trigger causes the small airways to become tighter and narrower, the lining begins to swell and for some, mucus builds up, narrowing the tubes even more. The result of these symptoms is that the sufferer finds it progressively difficult to breathe.

Asthma triggers

Each asthma sufferer will have a known trigger (something that irritates the airways and causes their symptoms) which is very specific to them; some people will have only one trigger, others may have several. In the outdoors triggers may include air pollutants, emotions (such as fear), exercise, food, pollen, certain medications and the weather. Most people with asthma learn to control their condition on a day to day basis by avoiding their known triggers and if necessary, taking prevention medication.

Medication

All known asthmatic people should have a reliever inhaler, which is usually blue and used to immediately relieve the symptoms of an asthma attack. The drug is breathed in and quickly relaxes the muscles around the narrowed airways, allowing the tubes to open wider thus making it easier to breathe.

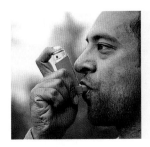

ASTHMA RELIEVER MEDICATION

During an attack the asthmatic person needs their reliever inhaler (usually blue). They cannot overdose on their reliever medicine. With high doses they can sometimes experience an increased heart rate, or on occasions, mild muscle shakes; however these generally wear off within a few minutes or a few hours at the most.

Asthma first aid

People with asthma learn to manage their condition and usually deal with their attacks without the need for any assistance. However on occasions the attack does not respond to reliever medication; perhaps because they waited too long to take their medicine, or some other complication such as a chest infection. Whatever the reason, when initial treatment is delayed, or simply doesn't work, the situation becomes worse, as the already narrowed tubes of the lower airway become swollen and even more constricted. This can severely affect breathing, which when combined with exhaustion, may cause the casualty to stop breathing.

LOOK OUT FOR

Early signs may include:

Tight chest and coughing.

Wheezing.   ...

Shortness of breath.

Difficulty in speaking, short sentences.

In a prolonged or severe attack you may also see:

Short sentences becoming one word answers. Eventually unable to speak.

Exhaustion.

Grey-blue colouring in skin, lips, ear lobes and nail beds.

Use of neck and upper arm muscles to help with breathing.

Casualty is confused, goes quiet and loses consciousness.

WHAT TO DO

Help the casualty to sit down.

Stay calm and reassure the casualty.

Encourage the casualty to use their reliever inhaler.

Kneel down, give them eye contact, encourage them to breathe slowly and deeply with you.

Encourage them to take their medication as required.

A mild attack should ease within a few minutes. If there is no improvement or you think this may be some other medical condition:

Dial 999/112 – request police – then ask for mountain rescue.

Insulate from the ground, provide shelter and monitor the vital signs; level of response (AVPU), breathing and pulse until help arrives.

Be prepared to start basic life support (CPR) if the casualty stops breathing.

REAL
LIFE
STORY

Asthma

Exertion from running or pushing myself too hard can cause me to start having an asthma attack, especially if I don't stop to regain my breath. I also seem to suffer when the weather is particularly cold and dry, or when I have a cough.

During an attack, the first thing I am aware of is a feeling of tightening in my chest; it can feel like my throat and lungs are burning. My breathing becomes much harder and I feel I have to take much bigger breaths, heave almost, really concentrating on just breathing in and out. You can hear me wheeze/gasp and maybe see that I am almost gulping, it really can be just so hard to get enough air.

With prolonged attacks the muscles around my ribcage will begin to ache, the harder it becomes to gain breath. It can feel like your throat is swollen, dry, and that you cannot get enough air into your lungs. My heart rate will rise as I struggle to breathe, and I may start to panic if I do not have my reliever medicine to hand. An attack can be very exhausting, as you have to put such a lot of effort into breathing.

I usually see a dramatic reduction in my symptoms (wheezing) within a few minutes of taking my blue reliever medication. If I have allowed the attack to continue before resorting to taking my inhaler, it may take a second dose to have any effect, as the more swollen the airways become the harder it is to get the medicine into the right spot. If all else fails (for instance if medicine is not having the desired effect, or if I do not have my reliever medicine with me) I need you to try and keep me calm, get me to focus on my breathing.

I may need assistance to walk (make sure I don't exert myself, so offer to carry rucksacks, etc). The right treatment at the right time can seem like a small miracle, so the sooner you can get some form of reliever medicine to me, the better.

Liz Giles

Those who call out mountain rescue for help with severe asthmatic attacks may have to wait some considerable time before that help arrives. Carrying an asthma reliever medication in an outdoor first aid kit is a sensitive issue. The law, as it stands in the UK, is very clear: this medication is a prescriptive drug for a named person only despite being on sale in supermarkets. There are very strict legal requirements that supermarkets must follow, which basically means you can't just turn up and buy one. I raised this matter with Asthma UK and, after a lengthy discussion, their opinion was as follows.

Reliever inhalers are prescribed for use by an individual person only. For that reason Asthma UK is legally unable to recommend the practice of using somebody else's reliever inhaler. However, in an emergency situation where the individual is having a severe asthma attack and their own reliever inhaler is not available, using another person's reliever inhaler is preferable to being unable to give any medicines.

Asthma UK

A common sense approach to this rather sensitive issue needs to be adopted. Many outdoor first aiders are of the opinion that if a person suffering a life-threatening severe attack in a remote setting can be saved by medication, then that medication should be made available.

Hyperventilation – panic attack

Hyperventilation is an increased breathing rate caused by some overwhelming emotional event, which may accompany a panic attack. Hyperventilation was once described to me as feeling like "the air wasn't getting right down into the bottom of my lungs", and that they were unable to completely fill their lungs.

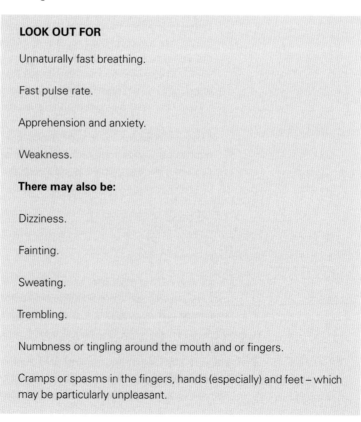

LOOK OUT FOR

Unnaturally fast breathing.

Fast pulse rate.

Apprehension and anxiety.

Weakness.

There may also be:

Dizziness.

Fainting.

Sweating.

Trembling.

Numbness or tingling around the mouth and or fingers.

Cramps or spasms in the fingers, hands (especially) and feet – which may be particularly unpleasant.

WHAT TO DO

Reassure the casualty, in a calm but firm manner.

Establish a history: have they ever had a panic attack before?

If possible remove them from the cause of the distress or anxiety.

Encourage or 'coach' the casualty to breathe more slowly.

Once recovered, the casualty may have a headache or feel shaky and weak.

If the casualty fails to recover, or you think this may be some other medical problem:

Dial 999/122 – request police – then ask for mountain rescue.

Insulate from the ground, provide shelter and monitor the vital signs; level of response (AVPU), breathing and pulse until help arrives.

The age old technique of placing a paper bag over the casualty's face is no longer recommended, as this may be dangerous if the casualty has an unrecognised lung problem. Simply use a firm, but caring manner to enable the casualty to regain control of their breathing.

Allergic reactions and anaphylaxis

Around 1–6% of the UK population are thought to be sensitive to latex. It may be prudent therefore to avoid placing latex gloves in your outdoor first aid kit, or carry other types as well, for example nitrile or vinyl.

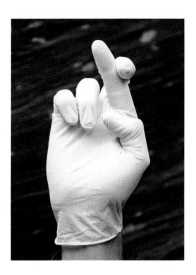

An allergy is when the body over-reacts to some foreign material (known as an allergen). In its mildest form an allergen can create a localised reaction in the area of contact. A severe response can result in the casualty going into anaphylactic shock causing breathing difficulties, and can be potentially fatal. The symptoms usually start between three and sixty minutes after contact with the allergen.

Causes of an allergic reaction

In reality **any** substance can cause an allergic reaction, but the more common triggers are food stuffs like peanuts or shellfish. However research indicates that in the remote setting triggers tend to be wasp or bee stings, or a bite from a snake.

Mild to moderate allergic reaction

Mild to moderate allergic symptoms are numerous and may occur in any order. It is also possible for them to progress rapidly from mild into severe.

Hives, also known as 'nettle rash', are pale red, raised, itchy lumps on the skin.
Photo:
www.istockphoto.com

LOOK OUT FOR

Symptoms vary; the casualty may show some of the following.

Mild early symptoms include:

Itchy skin.

Running eyes and nose.

Nettle rash (hives).

Moderate: as the reaction develops you may also see:

Swelling, particularly of the face.

Difficulty in swallowing or a feeling of a lump in the throat.

Tingling, itching or burning sensation in the mouth.

Wheezing and shortness of breath.

Anxiousness.

Abdominal pain, nausea and vomiting.

Treatment of any allergic reaction is to remove the allergen that is causing the problem, for example stop eating and remove the item from the mouth or remove insect sting from the skin. Further treatment may include medications such as oral antihistamines, or for skin reactions (over a small area) the application of a cold wet cloth, or ice (do not place ice directly onto the skin).

Severe allergic reaction – anaphylaxis

Generally the casualty will look and feel unwell. Most reactions happen over several minutes and the casualty is usually anxious and may experience 'a sense of impending doom'.

LOOK OUT FOR

Mild symptoms, progressing to include any of the following:

Throat and tongue swelling – the casualty may feel like the throat is closing up.

Increased breathing difficulties.

Feeling tired and weak.

Lowered level of response into unconsciousness.

Breathing and heart may stop.

The speed with which these signs and symptoms happen is unpredictable; those with a particular sensitivity can go into a severe reaction very quickly. If the casualty has a history of anaphylaxis they may have been prescribed an adrenaline (epinephrine) auto injector-pen by their doctor such as an EpiPen or Anapen.

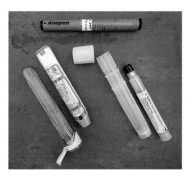

Here are some examples of auto-injectors. The green Anapen and the two EpiPens currently in circulation (the new type on the left, the old one on the right) with their carrying cases. Photo: Katherine Wills

WHAT TO DO

Act quickly, if possible remove the allergen.

Sit the casualty down.

Start your **ABC**s.   ...

Find out what happened. Is there a history of a common or known trigger?

If you find a life-threatening problem in your ABCs this is anaphylaxis.

Dial 999/112 – request police – then ask for mountain rescue.

The casualty **needs** adrenaline! Check if they are carrying their own medication – an auto-injector of adrenaline (epinephrine). If necessary assist them in using it: they are trained to inject into the outer thigh **only**, nowhere else.

If they have a wheeze or difficulty breathing and normally use an asthma inhaler, encourage them to use it. This casualty would benefit from taking oral antihistamines.

Keep the conscious casualty sitting up to help with breathing, place an unconscious casualty in a safe airway position and treat for shock.

Insulate from the ground, provide shelter and monitor vital signs; level of response (AVPU), breathing and pulse.

If the casualty stops breathing, be prepared to start basic life support (CPR).

REAL
LIFE
STORY

Living with anaphylaxis

The first sting shook me and I gripped my leg in a panic, at this point I felt dizzy. The second sting felt like it was going straight through my leg. Very quickly I felt my heart start to beat faster and then pound in my chest as if trying to burst out. I remember clutching my chest, the anxiety and fear was enormous, I felt my throat start to swell and I couldn't catch my breath. Eventually I passed out and I woke in hospital some time later with lumps and hives all over my arms and legs. Fortunately medics at the scene had recognised the symptoms as anaphylaxis, and administered adrenaline.

The next time I was stung my wife and I were walking in Snowdonia, and a bee stung me on my hand. Within sixty seconds I was experiencing the same symptoms as the previous attack and collapsed to the ground. On this occasion I didn't pass out but the antihistamines my doctor had prescribed were in the bottom of my rucksack and my wife had to empty the contents out, while I was still attached to it.   ...

Luckily two gentlemen came up the ridge, both doctors and helped, one having an EpiPen with him. After this attack I was prescribed my own EpiPen. I now carry two; if the first doesn't work within 15 minutes then we use the second. We also have a spare one in the kitchen which has proven to be very useful. One summer evening while carrying a tray of meat out for a BBQ I was stung by a wasp. I can remember my usual pounding heart and the shortage of breath. People were running towards me, then it all became a cascade of voices and I remember someone saying "he's having a heart attack".

My wife had rushed into the kitchen to get the spare EpiPen. On returning to the patio a number of people had started to treat me for a heart attack, because of my chest pain, and my poor wife had to fight her way past them to quickly inject me in the thigh.

Phil Hughes

Adrenaline

The immediate life-saving treatment for an anaphylactic reaction is an injection of adrenaline (epinephrine) and the sooner a casualty receives adrenaline, the better their chances of survival. There is no way of foreseeing the severity of an anaphylactic reaction; just because the casualty had a mild reaction previously does not mean future reactions will be the same.

Evidence suggests that delayed administration of adrenaline (e.g. waiting for mountain rescue or a helicopter winchman to administer it) greatly increases the risk of the casualty dying. The individual is taught how to administer their own auto-injector of adrenaline (EpiPen or Anapen). However, should the casualty be unable to administer it themselves, or they become unconscious before they are able to do so, you may be called upon to assist. The instructions are printed clearly on the side of the auto-injector; stay calm, read the information and follow the directions.

The effects of adrenaline are temporary; it is possible therefore, to see the symptoms return as the medication begins to wear off. Because of this, your casualty will need to be urgently evacuated to hospital.

OUTDOOR FIRST AID

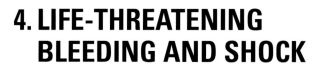

4. LIFE-THREATENING BLEEDING AND SHOCK

In simple terms, shock is a problem with the circulatory system – heart, blood vessels and blood – which results in insufficient oxygen reaching the body's tissues and vital organs. The most common reason for a casualty going into shock following an accident is life-threatening bleeding. The body can tolerate a certain amount of blood loss, however if bleeding is not stopped, the situation will eventually reach a critical point where the body can no longer cope and the whole system begins to fail. Shock is a true emergency and requires prompt first aid action and urgent evacuation.

Shock

The term 'shock' is generally misunderstood and often misused. Many people confuse it with the body's reaction to psychological stresses, such as surprise, grief, pain, distress, etc. Unfortunately, the symptoms are very similar and although psychological shock is unpleasant, it is not an emergency. Shock in its truest sense, however, is a life-threatening physical condition which, if not treated, will result in death.

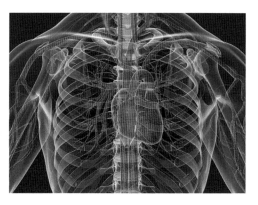

The circulatory system consists of the heart, the blood vessels (arteries and veins) and the blood. Photo: www.istockphoto.com

Shock is caused by one of three circulatory problems: a faulty pump (heart), the blood vessels becoming baggy (dilated), or the system leaking (blood loss). Shock is usually labelled according to what causes it, although the end signs and symptoms are often similar. If the heart fails the blood is no longer being pumped effectively around the body in order to send oxygen to the body's tissues; this is referred to as **cardiogenic shock**.

Another type of shock occurs when the arteries and veins become too dilated resulting in an insufficient amount of blood in the system to work effectively. This can happen with some spinal and head injuries – **neurogenic shock** – and also in a severe allergic reaction – **anaphylactic shock**.

The third type of shock, and the most common, is from massive blood loss – **hypovolaemic shock**. This can be caused by external bleeding which may be obvious or internal bleeding which is hidden inside the body. This chapter deals specifically with blood loss shock.

Blood loss shock explained

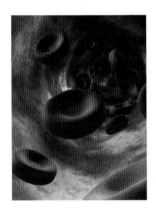

Photo:
www.istockphoto.com

As the body loses significant amounts of blood the tissue and organs become starved of oxygen and a message is sent to the heart to speed up. If the system continues to leak, the heart will need to beat increasingly faster in order to deliver sufficient amounts of oxygen to the tissue and organs. The heart doesn't just work in isolation, the blood circulating needs to take in oxygen (and get rid of carbon) through breathing. As the heart rate increases so does breathing.

At the same time a message is sent to the blood vessels feeding less important areas of the body, such as the gut, muscles and skin, telling them to constrict (become narrower), reducing blood flow. As this happens you may notice changes in skin colour and temperature; the casualty may start to look pale and feel cold. In the meantime the vital organs of the brain, heart muscle and kidneys continue to be fed with what little blood is still circulating; this combined with their own self-preservation mechanisms allows them to continue functioning for longer. The blood supply to the brain is protected right to the end. Eventually the part of the brain which controls consciousness becomes starved of oxygen and the casualty becomes increasingly anxious, agitated, confused, drowsy and ultimately unconscious.

The increase in heart rate and the amount of blood pumped, along with the faster breathing rate and the redirection of the precious blood to the vital organs of the heart, brain and kidneys, are the body's way of coping or 'compensating' for blood loss. However, if bleeding is not stopped, there is only a certain amount of time before the system begins to fail, the pump stops working and the casualty dies.

POTENTIAL LIFE-THREATENING BLEEDING INJURIES

Thigh bones – Break your thigh bone and if it remains **closed** (i.e. there is no tear in the skin over the break) you are likely to lose between 500ml and 1000ml of blood (0.88 and 1.75 pints). If **open** (i.e. there is a tear in the skin over the break) this can increase to between 1000ml and 2000ml (1.75 and 3.5 pints).

Pelvis – This can vary from a minor injury causing about 500ml of blood loss (0.88 pint), to major, causing you to lose **all** your blood.

Spleen, liver or chest injury – These can be trivial causing you to lose a few teaspoons of blood, or serious, causing you to lose **all** your blood.

Identifying blood loss shock

It is difficult to work out if someone is going into blood loss shock for two reasons; firstly it's virtually impossible to work out how much blood has been lost – either external and/or internal; secondly, certain casualties compensate incredibly well, even when they have significant blood loss and may initially appear fine.

You will need to rely on other factors to help you. Take a history, find out exactly what happened and consider the 'mechanisms of injury'. Look for significant and obvious external bleeding, as well as other injuries that may cause internal bleeds, such as a broken pelvis, broken thigh bones, chest injury or abdominal injury – or any combination thereof!

Establishing the mechanisms of injury – and the forces involved – will help you to assess the likelihood of certain types of injuries, and the potential for the casualty to go into shock.
Photo:
www.istockphoto.com

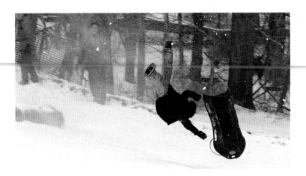

The severity of shock depends largely on how much and how quickly the casualty loses blood: usually the faster the blood loss, the more severe the signs and symptoms. Other factors may also interfere with how quickly the signs and symptoms of shock appear, including the casualty's age, fitness level, any pre-existing diseases or conditions and medications they may be taking.

Very young and old casualties will have differing abilities to deal with significant blood loss. The elderly, and those with chronic medical conditions, are less likely to cope due to their reduced physical reserve. They may also be taking certain medications, such as beta blockers, which will mask changes in the heart and breathing rates, or blood thinning drugs such as warfarin which will hamper blood-clotting.

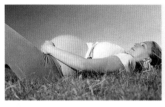

Photo:
www.istockphoto.com

PREGNANCY AND LIFE-THREATENING BLEEDING

Pregnant women nearing their term have an increased blood volume of up to 50% which means that even with severe blood loss, you may notice few signs or symptoms.

On the other hand children and those who are very fit and healthy will compensate and, despite considerable blood loss, at first appear fine. Eventually they reach a breaking point, when they can no longer cope, and catastrophically deteriorate.

Treating blood loss shock

Life-threatening bleeding and shock should be treated at the same time, not in isolation. Your aim should be to do some simple procedures, do them quickly, keep the casualty warm (hypothermic blood does not clot as well as blood at a normal body temperature) and arrange for the casualty to be evacuated to hospital. This is an emergency!

LOOK OUT FOR

In an adult:

Skin – pale, cold, sweaty.

Fast heart rate (over 100 beats per minute).

Fast breathing (over 20 breaths per minute).

Thirst.

Altered mental state – anxious, restless, confused, drowsy into unconsciousness.

WHAT TO DO

Dial 999/112 – request police – then ask for mountain rescue.

Treat external bleeding and identify possible internal bleeding such as into the chest, abdomen, or breaks to the pelvis or thigh bones.

Lie the casualty down.

Reassure and comfort the casualty.

Keep the head either level or slightly lower than the rest of the body.

If possible raise the legs, sending blood to the vital organs.

Keep the casualty warm, insulate from the ground.

Provide shelter and monitor the vital signs; level of response (AVPU), breathing and pulse.

To effectively treat blood loss shock, significant external bleeding needs to be stopped without delay. The standard and commonly recognised approach to first aid is to follow the **ABC** method: **A**irway, **B**reathing and then assess **C**irculation which includes treating catastrophic life-threatening bleeding. The **ABC** framework is designed to encourage you to concentrate, as a priority, on the importance of **A**irway and **B**reathing, and for good reason as this approach saves lives. However, if a casualty is losing life-threatening amounts of blood, it really won't matter what you do with the **A**irway or **B**reathing assessment because by the time you get round to checking and treating a problem like catastrophic bleeding, your casualty may well be dead.

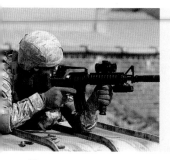

CATASTROPHIC LIFE-THREATENING BLEEDING

Military medics have found that external bleeding is the leading cause of combat death. Subsequently the UK military have changed the standard **ABC** of first aid to <**C**>**ABC** (where <**C**> stands for catastrophic bleeding). This new <**C**> **ABC** approach now forms the basis of the modern pre-hospital approach within the NHS, including most ambulance services.

Photo:

www.istockphoto.com

For a casualty who is conscious, that is they are talking, shouting or screaming, you can assume the **A**irway is open, and they are **B**reathing. The next logical thing to do therefore is to control the life-threatening bleed. With the unconscious casualty it may be possible to ask someone to assist in controlling catastrophic bleeding, while you quickly work through your **A**irway and **B**reathing checks – or perhaps you can manage them both at the same time.

However, you may decide on this **rare** occasion, to break away from the standard first aid **ABC** approach and control the catastrophic life-threatening bleed quickly, and then move onto your **A**irway and **B**reathing checks. This is a judgement call that you are going to have to make when faced with this situation. **Remember**: this is to control not just any bleed, but specifically obvious catastrophic life-threatening external bleeding.

Circulation checks

Your **C**irculation checks should include the following.

- Control any external bleeding.

- Recognise the **potential** for a casualty to go into blood loss shock, and urgently summon help.

- Identify other possible areas of internal bleeding.

- Make an assessment of skin colour, mental status and if possible find and take a pulse.

Controlling catastrophic life-threatening external bleeding

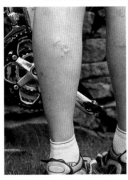

Photo: Katherine Wills.

There are two types of external bleeding that may be life-threatening; arterial which is usually bright red and 'squirts' out, and venous which is darker and usually dribbles or oozes out, except when large veins are involved, when it can flood out. Whether it is squirting or flooding doesn't really matter – just stop it!

VARICOSE VEINS

Varicose veins are swollen and enlarged veins and are very common. Those near the surface of the skin can sometimes bleed if they are caught and can be difficult to stop, particularly if the casualty is taking blood thinning medication such as warfarin.

WHAT TO DO

Your treatment will depend on where the wound is located and whether it is compressible.

Apply direct pressure over the top of the bleed.

If involving a limb elevate above the level of the heart.

If appropriate consider packing the wound, or using a haemostatic agent.

Apply a trauma dressing with compression bandage.

If necessary, as a last resort, consider a tourniquet.

Direct pressure and elevation above the heart

The vast majority of bleeding can be controlled by applying pressure **directly** over the wound and if possible, elevating above the heart (allowing gravity to help reduce the blood flow). Pressure can be applied by the fingers or hands (yours, the casualty's or a bystander's), a knee, a sterile dressing or any other improvised pressure dressing. Once you have controlled bleeding you can secure the dressing in place preferably using a compression band-age. For extremities, consider splinting; this will help to keep the dressing in place and stop any unnecessary movement which may trigger re-bleeding.

The key words here are **direct** and **pressure**: simply laying a dressing over the bleed is not applying direct pressure, and blood loss may simply continue to leak underneath the dressing. Remember, when an artery is involved, the spurting blood is under much greater pressure and this can make it much harder to stop.

Wound packing and haemostatic agents

If the wound is large or bleeding is in a non-compressible area (such as the groin, armpit or neck), it may be more appropriate to pack the wound with gauze and then place a dressing over the top.

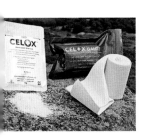

Haemostatic agents,
Celox granules and gauze.

Alternatively you can use a haemostatic agent, which is designed specifi-cally to stop bleeding. They are a relatively new concept within the civilian world, though developed and used significantly within military medicine. These novel haemostatic products include powders (that can be poured into wounds), special pads (that look like beer mats) and gauze impregnated with granular powder.

Compression trauma dressings (military)

Modern military compression trauma dressings have developed considerably over the years, many as a result of experiences within the battle field. Don't confuse these with simple wound dressings; they are very different. Compression dressings have additional elements: a thicker dressing pad and a strong elastic bandage capable of applying direct and significant pressure over the bleed.

Tourniquets

A tourniquet is a device used to cut off blood flow to a limb: by applying tight pressure around the arm or leg, it is possible to squash the blood vessels and stop blood travelling to the end of the limb. It can be used to stem catastrophic external life-threatening bleeding when all other treatments have failed. A tourniquet is a great life-saving piece of kit **if** it is used at the right time, with the right type of bleed, in the right way.

There is an awful lot of disagreement as to the appropriateness of using tourniquets. Indeed my research has highlighted how contentious this issue is among some medical authors of wilderness first aid books. Opinions vary from having 'no place at all', to its recognition as a rare but potentially life-saving technique.

Tourniquets have been thrust into the limelight over the last few years, not only as a vital piece of military medical kit in Iraq and Afghanistan, but also by their use in the civilian world from first aiders offering assistance to numerous casualties in the 7/7 London terrorist bombings.

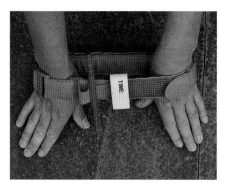

The Combat Application Tourniquet (CAT). This tourniquet is now carried by many ambulance services. It is used as a last resort to stem catastrophic life-threatening external bleeding.

Some would argue that the UK remote setting is unlikely to produce injuries similar to those found in terrorist incidents – specifically blast and/or penetrating injuries to limbs. However, significant falls down rock can, and do, leave casualties with multiple injuries, including traumatic near amputations of limbs.

Attempts should be made to stop the bleed by all other means before a tourniquet is considered. The only time this rule may be broken is if you need to control a catastrophic life-threatening bleed on a casualty who is trapped and the point of injury is out of reach, or with multiple casualties with extremity injuries such as in an explosion.

There is no getting away from the fact that there are potential risks associated with the use of tourniquets (including the loss of the limb), especially when you are unsure about what you are doing. However, there may be a few exceptional occasions when the application of a tourniquet may be necessary, even life-saving. Should you wish to consider this type of treatment, it is recommended that you attend a suitable first aid course and be instructed in its appropriate use and application.

Remember tourniquets are **only** used as a last resort and **only** with catastrophic life-threatening bleeding; less severe bleeds can be managed using simpler methods (see the chapter on **Care of Wounds**).

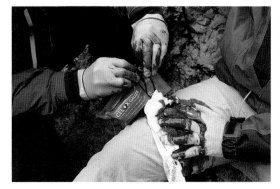

If significant bleeding is present (either internal or external) assume the casualty will go into shock, treat accordingly and urgently arrange for evacuation.
Photo: Brian Wills.

Identifying and treating other possible areas of bleeding

This check is to establish if there are other potential sites of less obvious life-threatening bleeding hidden inside the body. There are four areas that need to be considered including bleeding into the chest, the abdomen, or from breaks to the pelvis or thigh bones.

Bleeding into the chest may be picked up during your **B**reathing check (see the chapter on **Breathing Problems**). The abdomen should be visibly checked for any obvious wounds, swelling or bruising and gently palpated (felt with the hands and fingers) for any tenderness and/or swelling. The pelvis should **not** be physically examined or compressed. If conscious, the casualty may complain about pain in or around the pelvis; if unconscious, assume a pelvic fracture if the mechanism of injury involves significant forces. Fractured thigh bones must also be identified and treated.

Where a specific treatment is not indicated the advice is to keep the casualty calm and still; summon urgent help quickly; where possible insulate from the ground; provide shelter and monitor vital signs; level of response (AVPU), breathing and pulse while you await rescue.

Circulation assessment

This is a general assessment of how well the circulation is working. Firstly look at the casualty's skin colour; as shock develops the casualty will start off slightly pale, and then turn very pale, cold and sweaty. Another useful check is to assess their mental state. The casualty may initially be clear-headed and responsive, but then become anxious, restless, confused and eventually drowsy into unconsciousness. Finally taking a pulse can be a particularly valuable tool; the heart rate increases rapidly as shock develops. Monitoring and recording the pulse can provide you, and the rescue services attending, with useful baseline information.

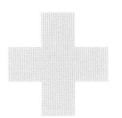

5. DRESSINGS AND BANDAGES

First aid kits contain a number of items, and the vast majority usually include some form of dressings and bandages. Ideally dressings should be shop-bought and sterile, as their purpose is to cover open bleeding or seeping wounds. Bandages on the other hand provide a number of different functions including securing dressings in place, providing support and stability for an injured joint or muscle, immobilising limbs or securing splints.

In the remote setting a first aid kit may not be readily available therefore you may have to improvise with whatever is to hand. Improvisation is an important part of remote first aid, and to do this successfully you need to understand the principles behind your treatment.

Dressings

There are numerous types of sterile dressings produced to deal with an assortment of wounds, from minor burns to a massive bleed. Here are some general principles to consider when applying a dressing.

WHAT TO DO

Sit the casualty down.

Put on your examination gloves.

Explain clearly what you are doing and if possible get the casualty involved.

If appropriate clean the wound and dry the surrounding skin (see chapter on **Care of Wounds**).

Choose a dressing appropriate to the type and size of the wound. ...

If you need to handle the dressing hold it by the edges and avoid touching the part that covers the wound.

Place the dressing directly over the top of the wound; don't slide it in from the side.

If the dressing does not have a bandage or adhesive strips, it will need to be secured using tape or a separate bandage.

Different types of dressings

Adhesive dressings

This group of dressings consist of a gauze or cellulose pad attached to an adhesive backing. Before applying make sure the wound is clean and the surrounding skin is dry. Ensure the casualty is not allergic to which ever adhesive product you use.

Plasters

Plasters are a piece of gauze stuck onto tape and used on small cuts and grazes. They can be bought in a variety of shapes and sizes, and made from a number of different materials, such as fabric or latex. Hypoallergenic plasters are available for those who are allergic to normal plasters and manufacturers also produce novelty designs for use on children.

Blister plaster

These are designed to stick to the damaged area producing a kind of 'second skin'. If applied early they can provide a barrier from friction, preventing a blister forming. They can also be applied directly onto blisters, and blisters that have torn open and are leaking. Designed to absorb moisture and create a protective cushion these specialised plasters can provide pain relief, protect against dirt or bacteria and encourage healing.

Blister plasters come in different shapes and sizes. Read the manufacturers instructions carefully.

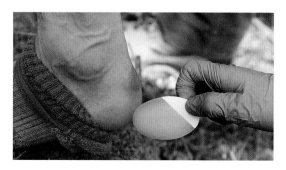

Wound closure strips

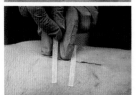

Most cuts do not include any loss of tissue, therefore the edges of the wound can be brought together; a bit like a jigsaw. This can then be held in place using specially made strips of tape, referred to as wound closure strips.

APPLICATION OF WOUND CLOSURE STRIPS

Dry the skin either side of the wound. If the casualty is excessively hairy it may be necessary to cut the hairs to ensure the tape sticks directly to the skin.

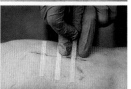

Place the first strip in the middle of the wound. Secure half the tape on one side and use your free fingers to push the opposite side of the wound closed, and then secure the other half of the tape. The edges of the wound should just gently touch – avoid pushing them too tightly together.

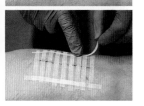

Repeat the process by placing your next strip between the first piece of tape and the end of the wound. The tape should extend 2–3cm beyond the wound on both sides.

Repeat until the wound is covered, leaving a 2–3mm gap between each strip.

A final 'locking' strip can be placed over the ends on both sides of the wound.

It is not recommended, as a precaution against risk of infection, to close animal or human bites, deep puncture wounds, deep wounds to the hands or feet, or wounds that contain crushed or damaged tissue.

Burn dressings

Minor burns can be dealt with using a non- or low-adherent wound dressing. A simple, easy and cheap alternative is to use cling film. As long as the first few centimetres are discarded, the cling film is sterile. Remember to use it as a dressing and place it over the burn; do not wrap around a burnt limb like a bandage as this will cause constriction if the injury swells. Cling film is protective, and soothes. It does not stick to the skin and has the added advantage of being transparent – allowing the burn to be assessed in hospital without the need for removal.

Low- and non-adherent wound dressings

These thin absorbent pads are used on wounds that are producing light to moderate amounts of leakage and are ideal for use on superficial abrasions, lacerations and minor burns. The different brands do vary but in essence they all draw the seepage away from the wound. Select the correct size of pad for the injury; this should extend well beyond the edges of the wound. When removing it from its package hold by the edges, and avoid placing your fingers on the area that will make contact with the wound. Once in place secure with tape or a bandage.

Low- and non-adherent wound dressings come in a variety of sizes.
Photo: Brian Wills

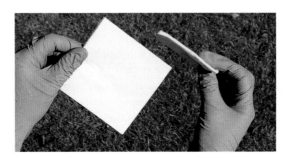

Unfortunately despite their name, some of these products have gained a reputation for actually sticking fiercely to the surface of the wound and surrounding skin, causing pain and damage to the wound on removal. More modern non-adherent dressings (such as those coated in silicone) are gaining popularity as they don't stick to the wound or surrounding skin. The drawbacks are they are not cheap and require a further dressing on top to hold them in place.

Wound dressings

These are dressing pads attached to a roller bandage and sealed in a protective wrapper. This popular dressing comes in a variety of sizes and is referred to by a number of different names including 'sterile wound dressing' and 'first aid dressing'.

When opened and unravelled the wound dressing has a short length of bandage, a dressing pad, and finishes with a longer section of bandage. The pad is placed directly over the wound and the bandage used to secure it in place.

APPLICATION OF A WOUND DRESSING

Break the plastic seal on the bandage and remove it from its packaging. Unwind the bandage until the dressing pad is exposed. Avoid touching the pad by holding the bandages either side.   ...

Lay the dressing pad directly onto the wound. Wrap the short bandage around the limb once to secure the dressing; if possible, ask the casualty to hold the short end out of the way.

Continue to wind the other end of the bandage around the limb, completely covering the wound dressing pad. Check with the casualty that the bandage is not too tight.

Keep the short end of the bandage free and finish by bringing the two ends of the bandage together and tie a knot. Finally check circulation beyond the bandage to make sure it is not too tight.

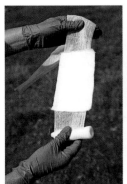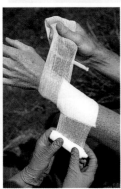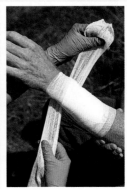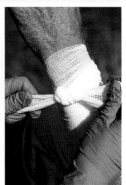

Compression trauma dressings (military)

'The emergency bandage – trauma wound dressing' is the current NATO/British Army issue trauma wound field dressing. Accidents in the mountains do sometimes result in significant injuries which may require more than just a standard wound dressing.

This bandage (also known as an 'Israeli bandage or dressing') comes in two sizes; 4 and 6 inch. It has a substantial dressing pad with a heavy duty elasticated compression bandage attached and is designed to stop all types of bleeds from minor to catastrophic. It is possible to buy this product with or without a small plastic pressure bar (the bandage can be fed back into it and used to generate more pressure). The end of the bandage is secured in place by a plastic bar with grab hooks at either end.

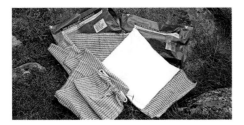

The emergency bandage – trauma wound dressing.

Haemostatic dressings and products

Haemostatic products have been developed to control emergency bleeding and used with great success within the military setting. The products are available in a number of different forms, including a granular powder (which is poured into the wound), a dressing (or pad) and gauze impregnated with the clotting agent. Common brand names include Celox, HemCon and QuickClot.

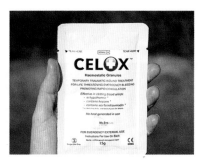

Celox can be used to stem catastrophic life-threatening bleeds and will work on cold (hypothermic) casualties as well as those who are taking blood-thinning drugs such as warfarin.

Airtight dressing

This dressing does not allow air to pass through it. It is used on open chest wounds when the injury is big enough to allow air to enter directly into the chest through the wound. Specific airtight dressings can be bought. However, it is possible to improvise using cling film, or the inside of the cellophane packaging from a standard wound dressing. Simply open the packaging – avoid touching the inner cellophane – cut to size, apply directly over the wound, then tape on **three** sides leaving one side open (see the chapter on **Breathing Problems**).

Improvised dressings

Dressings are placed directly onto an open wound to help keep it clean, prevent infection, absorb blood or wound leakage, encourage healing and protect from any further damage or harm. An 'ideal' wound dressing should be sterile, breathable, control leakage and provide a moist and healing environment. Improvised dressings may not fulfil all these requirements; however, they may temporarily provide some of them.

From my own experience a number of rescues in the mountains have shown first hand just how creative first aiders can be; socks used to stem a bleeding wrist, rolled up T-shirts to stop bleeding scalps, sanitary towels used as emergency dressings and secured in place with duct tape. Few, if any, of these can be considered 'sterile', however they were successful to one degree or another, in stopping bleeding and/or protecting the wound from further harm.

REAL
LIFE
STORY

Photos: Kat Spinney

Improvised dressing

Sam, Neil and I were four hours into our walk and were scrambling through a boulder field with massive blocks of rock. As I stepped up, my lower foot slipped down slightly. Unfortunately, my shin had been right next to a sharp-edged rock which cut a big four inch slice across my shin. I didn't fall over or lose balance so when I looked down I was surprised to be able to see inside my leg! I noticed there was something dark inside which I took to be dirt (but I think it was the muscle I could see), so I just clamped my hand straight over it to hold it together and said something like "guys ... I think you had better come back down".

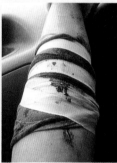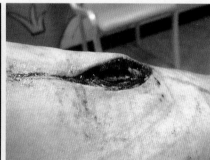

Neil got our group shelter out while Sam took a look, then they flushed it through with water from our CamelBak (a brand of water container). Sam wrapped his Buff (a kind of multifunctional tubular headgear) around the wound while Neil looked for an evacuation route. Neil had some tape so Sam taped over the Buff to keep it in place and I put on my long trousers to try to protect it further. Fortunately I was able to crawl out of the boulder field and, with a little help, made it back to the road. We were lucky to get a lift back to our car and finished the day with an unplanned visit to the hospital.

Kat Spinney

Bandages

Bandaging is a relatively simple procedure and can provide the first aider with a multitude of treatment options; including holding dressings in place or supporting a joint or muscle injury. Here are some general principles to consider when applying a bandage.

WHAT TO DO

Dress all wounds.

Select the correct type and size of bandage depending on what you are trying to achieve (i.e. secure a dressing or support an injured joint).

Work from the front of the casualty on the side of the injury. Avoid having to lean across their body.

Ask the casualty to support the injured part.

Apply bandages firmly, but not too tight; constantly check with the casualty.

Try to avoid excessive creases or gaps between each wrap of the bandage.

If possible, leave fingers and toes exposed, allowing for circulation checks.

When finished, secure the bandage in place.

Check circulation in the area beyond a bandage and monitor often.

Checking circulation after bandaging

It is good practice after applying a bandage to check it is not too tight. If the casualty complains of pins and needles or numbness beyond the bandage, take it off and re-apply (without disturbing the dressing). For the unconscious casualty check circulation by doing a **capillary refill test**. Press on the skin or nail bed for five seconds and then release (it will go pale); the colour usually returns in about two seconds. If it takes longer, then either circulation may be compromised, or the casualty may simply be cold; if unsure test on the other limb to compare.

Capillary refill test.
Photos: Brian Wills

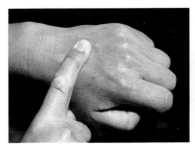
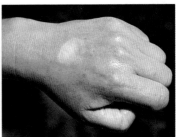

Different types of bandage

There are three main types of bandage: roller, tubular and triangular.

Roller bandages

Roller bandages are made from a number of different materials including gauze, elastic fabric, cotton or linen. There are three basic types of roller bandage: open-weave, elastic adhesive, and crepe.

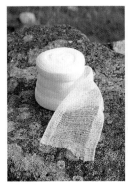

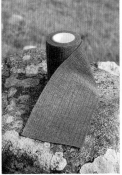

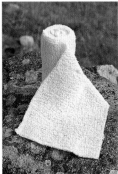

Open weave bandage – used to secure a dressing in place.

Elastic adhesive bandage – sticks to itself but not to skin. Firm support for muscle and joint injuries.

Crepe bandage – used for treating sprains and strains, and securing a dressing or splint in place

Application of a roller bandage

This simple spiral method of applying a roller bandage is used on cylindrical body parts such as an arm, leg, etc. Keep the rolled 'body' of the bandage uppermost so that it unwinds easily, and avoid dropping it.

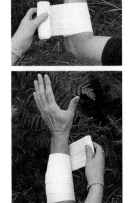

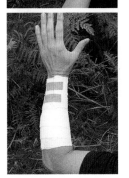

SPIRAL TECHNIQUE

Place the end of the bandage (tail) below the injury and wrap the bandage around twice to secure the tail in place.

Working up the limb wind the bandage in spiralling turns. Cover half to two thirds of the previous wrap with each new turn.

Finish the bandage off with one final straight turn then secure in place.

Bandaging – specific areas

SCALP

Place a dressing over the scalp wound.

Take a crepe bandage or equivalent and starting from the back of the head lay it loosely over the dressing to the casualty's eye brows and bring it back over.

With your free hand take hold of both layers of bandage at the back and ask the casualty to do the same at the front. Ask the casualty to pull the bandage towards their chin. At the same time you must pull both layers of bandage downwards at the back.

Maintaining the tension, start to wind the bandage around the head, keeping it level with the eye-brows at the front and low at the back of the head.

After a couple of wraps ask the casualty to let go of the front and at the same time you must let go at the back. Take hold of the flap at the front and lift it clear of the eyes and catch it with another wrap of the bandage. Do the same at the back. Once finished secure the bandage in place.

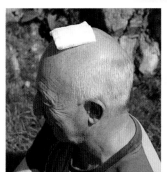 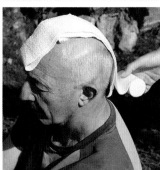 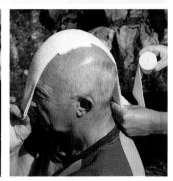

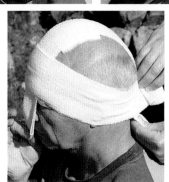 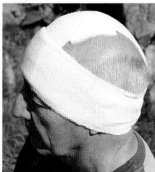

Photos: Brian Wills

HAND

Start with the tail of the bandage on the inside of the wrist. Make two complete wraps to secure the tail in place.

From the inside of the wrist pass the bandage diagonally across the back of the hand to the nail of the little finger, then across the front of the fingers.

Bring the bandage around to the back of the hand and pass it diagonally to the outer side of the wrist. Take the bandage around the wrist and back to the inner side under the thumb.

Repeat the figure-of-eight turns. Each new wrap of the bandage covers about two-thirds of the previous wrap. Once the hand is completely covered secure in place.

Photos: Brian Wills

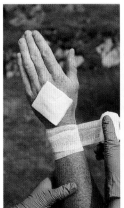 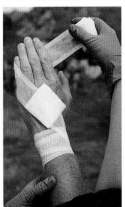 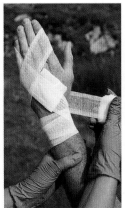 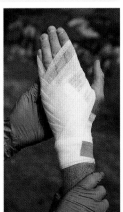

ELBOW OR KNEE

Support the injured limb in a position most comfortable for the casualty, with the joint slightly bent. Place the end of the bandage (tail) on the inner side of the joint and wrap the bandage around the actual joint twice to secure the tail in place.

Pass the bandage above the joint, wrapping it around the limb and covering the upper section of the initial secured tail wrap.

Bring the bandage over and around the lower part of the joint again covering the lower section of the initial tail wrap.   ...

Continue to pass the bandage above and below the initial tail wrap, in a figure-of-eight. Each new wrap covers about two thirds of the previous wrap. When finished secure in place.

Photos: Brian Wills

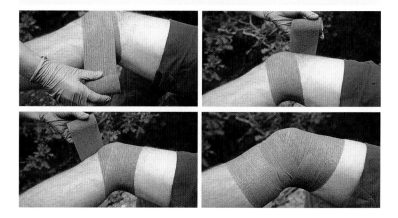

ANKLE

If available, apply a horse-shoe shaped piece of thin padding around the ankle. You can improvise with the pad of a wound dressing.

Start the bandage just above the toes and work toward the ankle covering the whole foot. Take the bandage around the back of the heel securing the bottom of the padding in place.

Bring the bandage back around the foot and then up and around the ankle in a figure-of-eight.

Repeat, covering the whole foot working up the ankle.

Finish mid-way up the calf and secure in place.

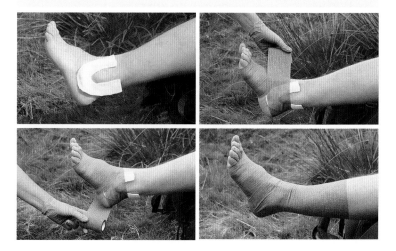

These bandaging techniques have been presented here to show you the correct methods of application. In reality bandages do not necessarily have to look 'pretty', they simply have to do the job for which they were intended. This is particularly so when improvising bandages from other pieces of kit or equipment.

Securing a roller bandage

Some bandage packs, such as crepe, contain little clips or safety pins, while others will require tape, or simply tuck the end in. Self-adhesive support bandages stick to themselves.

Adhesive tape

Bandage clips

Safety pin

Tuck in

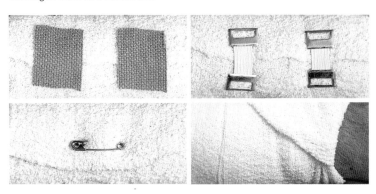

Tubular bandages

Tubular bandages are a seamless tube-like fabric which varies in thickness and elasticity. They can be used to secure dressings or to support injured limbs. The downside with tubular bandages is they come in a variety of sizes for a number of different body parts; you may not be carrying the correct size or type for your particular casualty.

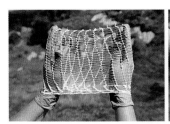
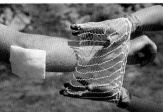
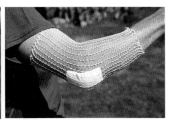

TUBULAR BANDAGE TO SECURE A DRESSING

These products are designed to hold a dressing in place, but do not apply significant pressure directly onto the wound.

Use your hands to open up the elasticated mesh bandage.   …

Keeping the mesh clear of the limb, slide the bandage up into position over the dressing.

Slowly remove your hands allowing the bandage to hold the dressing in place.

Tubular bandages for support are made from cotton with spirals of elastic woven into it and offers support for sprains and strains. Its use appears to have lost favour over the years; however within a first aid context, if in the short term it allows your casualty to evacuate themselves from the remote environment, some would argue it has a use.

Triangular bandages

This versatile triangle-shaped bandage can be used for many different purposes. Taken immediately out of its sterile pack it can be applied directly onto a wound as a dressing; when opened up it can be used as a sling for an arm (either elevated or standard arm sling). It can also be folded to create broad- or narrow-folded bandages, and used to secure dressings or immobilise and support a broken limb.

ELEVATED AND ARM SLING

The elevated sling secures the hand high up on the shoulder. It is useful for injuries to the hand and forearm, or where the casualty finds elevating the hand more comfortable. The arm sling can be used for injuries to the shoulder, upper arm, elbow, forearm and wrist. It may assist in easing pain from a rib fracture by supporting the arm.

For both the elevated and arm sling start by tying a simple over-hand knot in the 'point end' of the triangular bandage. This creates a small 'cup' for the elbow and avoids the need for a safety pin or tape.

Tie a knot in the 'point' end.

Triangular bandages are commercially produced in a sterile pack and usually contain safety pins or small clips. The size and quality of fabric varies according to the brand.

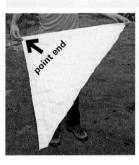
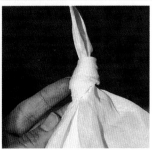

point end

ELEVATED SLING

Ask the casualty to place the injured arm across the body with the fingers touching the opposite shoulder. Support the elbow with the other hand.

Place the bandage over the injured arm keeping the knot at the elbow and the surplus bandage below.

Tuck the surplus bandage under the injured arm all the way down to the elbow.

Make two twists of the bandage close to the elbow to 'lock' it in place.

Take the bandage across the casualty's back to the top of the shoulder where the fingers are resting. Secure the bandage with a knot.

The finished sling should keep arm elevated and the hand high on the shoulder.

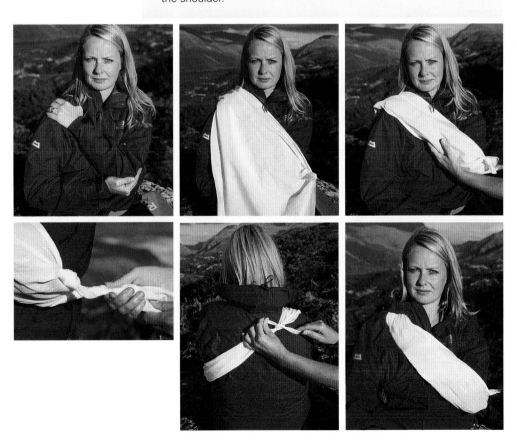

ARM SLING

The injured arm should be supported with the hand slightly higher than the elbow.

Feed one end of the bandage through the gap in the crook of the elbow and the body, keeping the knot at the elbow. Feed the end across the chest to the opposite shoulder.

Gently work the bandage across the chest towards the hand.

Bring the lower half of the bandage up and over the injured arm towards the other shoulder.

Secure the bandage with a knot to the side of the neck and if necessary pad underneath for comfort

Check your bandage from the front and ensure that the injured arm is either horizontal or slightly elevated at the hand.

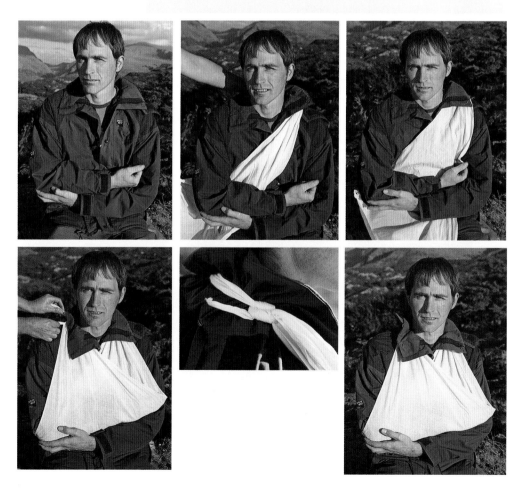

If the casualty is wearing a waterproof jacket, ensure the knot is placed under the hood. If the casualty needs to carry a rucksack, apply the sling while they are wearing it.

Broad- and narrow-folded bandages

By folding a triangular bandage you can create a broad or narrow bandage which can be used as a tie or strap. Find somewhere out of the wind. Open the triangular bandage out and rest it on your knee. Try to avoid placing it on the ground.

BROAD- AND NARROW-FOLDED BANDAGES

Fold the bandage in half so the point of the bandage touches the centre of the longest edge.

Fold the bandage in half again in the same direction (broad bandage).

Repeat the fold one final time (narrow bandage).

Photos: Brian Wills

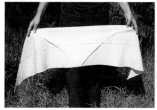 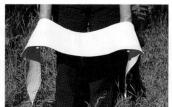 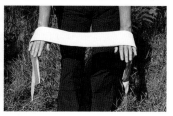

FOLDED BANDAGE: SECURING SLINGS

Add support to a sling by securing the arm further using a broad-folded bandage around the chest and sling, secured under the opposite armpit. Ensure the broad-folded bandage is above or below any fracture site, and not over it.

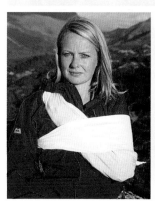 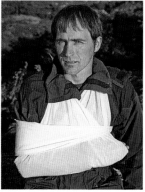

FOLDED BANDAGES: SECURING LEGS

Slide a narrow-folded bandage under the ankles to tie the feet together. Use broad-folded bandages to secure the ankle and knee joints. If available, a further broad bandage can be used to secure above the knees. Place plenty of padding between the knees and ankles

Start by securing the feet using a figure of eight. Bring the edges of the triangular bandage up, cross them over the front of the feet then take them around the boots and tie in the middle.

Secure the broad bandages by knotting away from the injured side; this is best achieved by tying in the middle, avoiding pressure points on the good leg. Monitor for swelling, and be prepared to loosen the ties if necessary.

Photos: Brian Wills

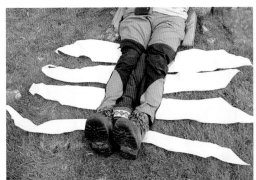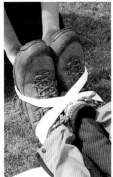
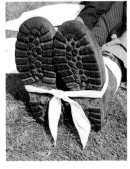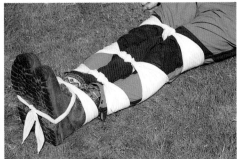

Improvised bandages

Depending on what you are trying to achieve, you may find a multitude of things that may temporarily do the job. A roller bandage can be improvised from a T-shirt (or other item of clothing) by cutting a strip of material.

IMPROVISED ROLLER BANDAGE

Lay the T-shirt out flat. Estimate the width of your bandage then mark a cutting line onto the T-shirt.Cut the T-shirt into the length of bandage you need. This could also be used as an improvised broad bandage by varying the width.

Photos: Brian Wills

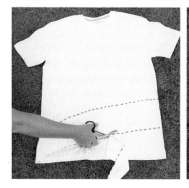 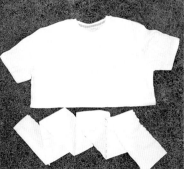

Improvised broad- and narrow-folded bandages can be used as ties to hold dressings in place, or to secure a fractured limb, or to hold a splint in position. Anything that can be used as a tie will work including sleeves of clothing, climbing equipment, parts of a rucksack, even bike inner tubes. Duct tape can be used as a tie by rolling it out then folding it back on itself so that the sticky sides adhere to each other. Be cautious with duct tape; its over en-thusiastic use when dealing with injuries can end up doing more harm than good, as it sticks fiercely to skin and is horrible to pull off an injured limb.

REAL
LIFE
STORY

Improvised splint – mountain biking

"What's the worst that can happen?" Those were Steve's words of wisdom as we took off down the trail. Old enough to know better I gave in to peer pressure and hit a fairly large jump, the first time out on a new bike. Too much speed and not enough skill led to me and the bike parting company, and me using a small tree to stop myself. Unfortunately my leg didn't want to stop and carried on going. The end result was a broken right thigh bone. When I came to rest my right leg was bent around the tree by about 45 degrees. Not a pretty sight!

Once the guys had stopped laughing and I had straightened my leg they set about getting me back onto the track and in a comfortable position. With no real first aid kit the lads went into improvisation overdrive; their ties were a couple of inner tubes and the padding was provided by a CamelBak. ...

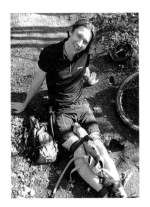

Photo: Steve Gouch

When this was in place they lifted me back onto the track where we waited for the paramedics to arrive. I was lucky enough to be with a fairly sensible group of guys who had a good practical knowledge of first aid and I was kept comfortable and cheerful until the paramedics arrived on the scene. They were suitably impressed with the makeshift splint to the point that they decided to leave it in place until they got me into the ambulance where they replaced it with a traction splint in an attempt to pull the bones back into alignment.

Three months rest and relaxation, plus a massive nail through my thigh bone and four cross pins, and I was back on the bike and haven't looked back since. The "worst" didn't happen. It could have been my head, pelvis or back that hit the tree!

Paul Greenwood

IMPROVISED SLINGS

Fleece/jumper – Fold the bottom of the fleece upwards to create either an elevated or arm sling secure with two large safety pins.

Orange survival bag – Cut an orange survival bag to size and use as you would a triangular bandage.

Belt or climbing sling – Feed the arm through the loop then take the sling (or belt) around the back of the neck and finish by placing the hand in the other loop. For an elevated sling secure around the wrist then fasten at the back of the neck ('collar-and-cuff'). Use plenty of padding to avoid pressure points.

Long-sleeved shirt/jumper – This can be used for either an elevated or arm sling. Place the injured arm in the position required, then secure at the cuff with a large safety pin.

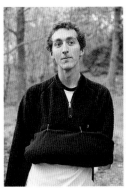
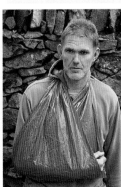
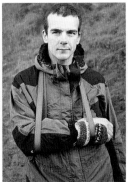
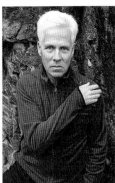

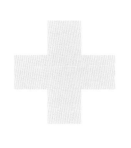

6. CARE OF BURNS

Burns usually involve the skin and the tissue beneath. On occasions, however, they may also affect the eyes, internal organs (from a lightning strike) and the airway. We burn ourselves in a number of ways including exposure to heat, friction, electricity, chemicals and radiation from the sun. In the remote setting burns can be caused by accidents around camp fires, cooking stoves and incidents in mountain bothies, as well as by lightning strikes or sunburn.

SKIN

Human skin has three basic layers. The top layer has different thicknesses according to where it is on your body; skin on the soles of feet is thicker than on the back of hands. It has many functions including protecting the body from infection and helping to regulate body temperature.

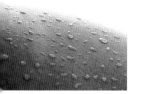

Photo:
www.istockphoto.com

Severity of a burn

Unless you witnessed the accident it is vital you take a history of what exactly happened. Consider the source of the burn, its temperature, and how long the casualty was exposed to it. The seriousness of a burn will depend on a number of things; primarily how deep the burn is (**burn depth**) and how much of the body has been burnt (**extent of burn**). Once you have answered these questions, think about the **location** of the burn; certain areas of the body cause more concern than others. Consider the possibility of **other injuries** and also the casualty's **age** and **general health**.

Burn depth

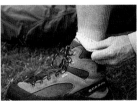

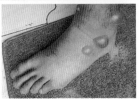

Burns are categorised according to the depth of damage. Superficial thickness (minor), partial thickness (moderate) and full thickness (serious). A single burn can have various depths; for example the centre of the burn may be full thickness with a ripple effect outwards into partial thickness and beyond into superficial.

Photo: Ben Buchanan

BURN DEPTH

Superficial burn – This involves the top layer of skin only. The skin looks red, and feels tender and painful but does not blister.

Partial thickness burn – Partial thickness burns extend deeper into the skin. These can be quite painful involving swelling and often a blister.

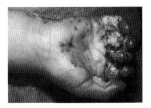

Full thickness burn – These are deep, including all layers of the skin and extend into the tissue below. The skin itself is numb, may appear black and charred or leathery white or pearly grey. There is no pain due to nerve damage. **Full thickness burns should be seen in hospital.**

Photo: Dr I Jones

Extent of burn

To work out how large the burn is you can use the 'rule of palm'. This method uses the size of the casualty's hand print (palm, fingers and thumb) as approximately 1% of that casualty's total body surface area – remember use the casualty's palm, not yours! The burnt area is expressed as a percentage of the casualty's total body surface area.

Rule of palm – only measure skin that is blistered or worse; do not include the simply reddened skin in your calculation.

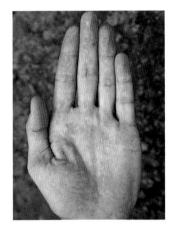

Location of burn

Unless extremely superficial or small, burns to the face, hands, feet or genitalia are considered serious, as are any burns that extend all the way around the chest, neck or a limb (circumferential), and any burn to the airway or eyes.

Face, eye and airway burns

Flame burns to the face, unless they are minor, should lead you to suspect a possible airway injury and the potential for the casualty to develop breathing difficulties. This is particularly so when the accident involves fire in an enclosed area. These casualties need careful and continuous monitoring (see the chapter on **Breathing Problems**).

Flame burns to the eyes usually go hand in hand with burns to the face. The natural reaction is to close the eyes and therefore the damage is often to the eyelid. Cover both eyes with a sterile dressing moistened with saline or drinking water. This is a serious injury which requires urgent medical attention.

Burns to hands and feet

Burns to the hand are common and most are small, relatively minor, and can be dealt with safely in the remote setting. However due to the functional importance of the hands and feet burns to these areas should be treated cautiously; if you are unsure evacuate the casualty urgently.

The general treatment for burns is to cool them by running under cold water for between ten and no longer than twenty minutes, and then cover them with an appropriate dressing. For extensive or significant burns to the hands or feet, once cooled, consider inserting them inside a polythene bag, such as a clinical waste bag: ask the casualty to keep the fingers or toes apart.

Genitalia

This area includes between the legs, around the anus and sex organs; usually seen as part of a larger injury to the trunk of the body and the legs, often as a result of a flame burn. In the remote setting however there always exists the possibility of an isolated scald injury from a hot drink spilt into the crotch.

Circumferential burns

A circumferential burn refers to any burn that encircles the neck, torso or a limb (such as an arm or a leg). A burn around the neck or chest can compress the tissue to such an extent that the casualty is unable to breathe and so the injury can be life-threatening. Circumferential burns around a limb may cut off the blood supply reaching the hands or feet which could be limb-threatening. These burns are an emergency and the casualty needs to be urgently evacuated to hospital.

Other injuries

While fleeing the source of a burn a casualty may fall, jump or trip, therefore it is important to assess the casualty thoroughly. You must perform a full **ABC** assessment as these 'other injuries' may be more serious than the burn itself.

Age of the casualty

Burns suffered by children (under 5 yrs old) or the elderly should be treated with extreme caution: the very young and old are more likely to experience complications. They do not tolerate the body's response to burns very well and are particularly prone to infection. It is also easy to accidentally over-cool the young and elderly. Ideally the water used to cool the burn should be tepid or lukewarm; however this may be a challenge in the remote environment. Remember cool the burn but keep the casualty warm.

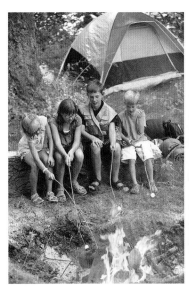

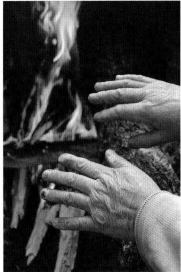

Young children (under 5) have little control over their environment, and their perception of danger is less: their ability to escape a burning situation may also be limited. Photo: www.istockphoto.com

Generally speaking the elderly have a reduced ability to heal and less physical capacity to cope with a burn injury. Photo: www.istockphoto.com

General health

The general health of a casualty plays a significant part in how well they cope with any injury but particularly a burn. Certain pre-existing medical conditions (such as heart, lung or liver disease, as well as diabetes, and even pregnancy) will influence how serious a burn is considered. If your casualty has poor circulation (as seen in Raynaud's disease), a weakened immune system (for example HIV or AIDS), or they are receiving chemotherapy treatment for cancer, they may also experience complications.

Complications

Burnt skin loses the ability to protect, which in turn increases the risk of infection. It is important therefore that you make every effort to keep the wound clean. If on expedition in the remote setting, monitor for signs of infection (see the chapter on **Care of Wounds**) and, if necessary, evacuate your casualty and seek further medical assistance.

Another complication arising from a serious burn (more than 10% on a child and 15% on an adult) is shock, resulting in insufficient oxygen reaching the body's tissue. This type of shock occurs due to the significant amounts of bodily fluid lost into the damaged tissue, and can kill (see the chapter on **Life-threatening Bleeding and Shock**).

Photo:
www.istockphoto.com

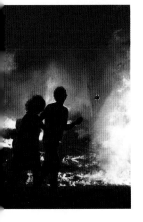

* **S** = Signs and symptoms
A = Allergies
M = Medications
P = Past medical history
L = Last meal
E = Events; what happened

TOP TIPS

If you require the assistance of the mountain rescue it would be useful to gather the following additional information.

What time did the burn occur?

What was the source of the burn, for instance flame, scald?

If involving flames, was the casualty in a confined space, or were they asleep at the time?

Has the casualty lost consciousness at any time?

Has the casualty any other injuries?

Is the casualty complaining of any pain?

Take a brief medical, allergy and drug history (*SAMPLE).

Types of burn

Contact with a hot
belay device.
Photo: Brian Wills

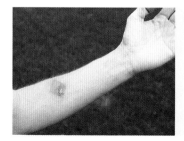

The following is a guide to different types of burn. The seriousness of the injury will depend on the factors mentioned previously. You will need to decide whether you are able to deal with this injury in the remote setting and self-evacuate, or whether you require urgent medical assistance and the attendance of mountain rescue.

CONTACT BURN

These burns occur when the skin comes into contact with a hot object, such as metal, hot coals or burning embers.

The injury will depend on the nature and temperature of the hot object, and the length of time of the contact.

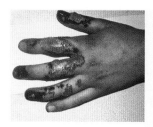

FLAME BURN

This type of burn involves fire. The flame may set light to clothing which can either ignite or melt onto the skin, giving a contact burn.

The depth of a flame burn is normally partial or full thickness.

Burns from a firework.
Photo: Dr I Jones

If the accident happened in an enclosed area, there is also a risk of an airway injury from inhaling hot air or smoke.

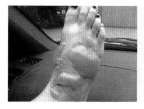

SCALD

These are the second most common burn injury types, and the most common in children. They are caused by hot liquids such as water or oil, or more commonly by steam.

Accident with camping
stove on expedition.
Photo: Richard Kimpton

WHAT TO DO

Check for any dangers to you and your casualty.

If the casualty is on fire tell them to drop to the floor and roll. Help by dousing them with water or use items of clothing to smother the flames.

Remove clothing over the burn; this can retain heat and continue the burning process. **However** do **not** remove any clothing that is stuck to the skin.

...

Remove rings, watches and any other items from around the burn, to avoid any restriction caused by tissue swelling.

Cool the burn quickly by placing it in running water from a stream, or failing that any source of clean water. Continue cooling for between ten and no longer than twenty minutes.

If necessary cover the burn with a suitable dressing (e.g. cling film).

In the case of a serious burn:

Dial 999/112 – request police – then ask for mountain rescue.

Insulate from the ground, provide shelter and monitor vital signs: level of response (AVPU), breathing and pulse, while awaiting rescue.

TOP TIPS

Do not burst any blisters from a scald, flame or contact burn.

Cooling will stop the burn getting worse therefore it is **critical** that you cool with water as quickly as possible; don't delay!

Don't use iced water as it can make the burn worse.

Cool the burn but keep the casualty warm; avoid hypothermia.

Don't apply adhesive tape to the skin: it is not always clear how far the burn extends. Tape accidentally applied to burnt skin will rip the skin when removed.

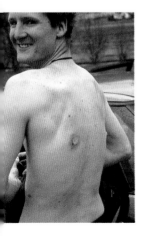

Dan was struck in the back by lightning. Photo: Jan Coggins

LIGHTNING WOUND

Lightning is a very short but explosive direct current electrical discharge associated with thunder storms.

The most common injury is through a direct hit and is often fatal. A 'splash effect' happens when lightning strikes another object (i.e. a tree) and then seeks the path of least resistance through the casualty. Contact with a conductive material (e.g. an ice axe) can also cause injury, as well as the explosive force of the strike. If the casualty is close to the direct strike it is possible for injury to occur from the ground current, which spreads outward from the point of contact – like ripples when you throw a stone into a pond.

In some cases a strike will stop both breathing and the heart.

WHAT TO DO

Check for any dangers to you and your casualty.

Follow your **ABC** approach.

Unconscious:

Dial 999/112 – request police – then ask for mountain rescue.

Casualty is breathing - continue with **C**irculation checks then a secondary survey for any injuries, place in a safe airway position.

Casualty is **not** breathing – start basic life support (CPR).

Conscious

Check for and treat any injuries; if possible evacuate the casualty and seek further medical assistance.

If their injuries are incapacitating, you will require assistance.

Dial 999/112 – request police – then ask for mountain rescue.

Insulate from the ground, provide shelter and monitor vital signs: level of response (AVPU), breathing and pulse, while awaiting rescue.

TOP TIPS

Casualties struck by lightning do not hold a charge! It is safe to touch them.

A person struck by lightning may not even realise they have been struck, they can have a reduced level of response, be confused and have memory loss.

If the casualty has been thrown a distance, consider the possibility of broken bones or a spinal injury – treat accordingly.

Sometimes they have a loss of sensation in the legs.

Any casualty struck by lightning should be seen at hospital – even if they look ok!

Lightning strike

With a dark pall menacing the lochs to the south and watery spring sunshine touching the summit snow of higher peaks to its north, a route called The Cobbler seemed to straddle the boundary between fair weather and foul. Swaddled as if for winter climbing we scrambled up the Southeast Ridge of South Peak; an easy mountaineering route that suited the day's mood. A continuation along The Arête led towards Centre Peak, the mountain's high point. While Jan led the final tower, he was unaware of an ugly wall of cloud cruising our way. Sleet fell in earnest as we coiled ropes on the sharp summit block. We slipped onto the descent route, a narrow ledge cutting across a face to a little tunnel and easy ground.

The ledge offered the best chance of shelter so here we perched, pleased to have found the only dry patch. As Jan reached over to offer a cup of soup there was a sudden almighty bang, a tremendous jolt that threw us both into the air – though fortunately not off the edge. My ears rang, my heart raced; the drink had vaporised. I must have been dazed. Was it a bomb, I wondered, or a curious case of exploding minestrone? Jan was quicker off the mark, strongly suggesting that we ought to get moving. My whole body buzzed with a sort of **funny bone** tingle, only rather more so; my limbs seemed to belong to someone else. We hobbled our way to lower ground, babbling in disbelief. We'd just been struck by lightning.

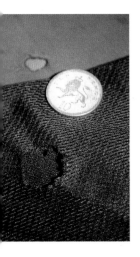

The burn holes through Dan's clothing. Photo: Dan Bailey

I noted a faint burning smell, a blend of singed polyester and barbecue; it was coming from me. But since we were both mobile damage assessments could wait. In mortal terror of further strikes we headed down as quickly as we could manage, my co-ordination soon returning. There had been no warning, no preceding rolls of thunder, no hair-raising buzz; just this single strike. Back at the car I peeled off layers, each one pierced with a sort of melted bullet hole. What we took to be the lightning's entry point on my back was a seared circle of odd-coloured concentric rings, like a target. That it gave me no pain at all I took to be a bad sign, but I could at least feel the scatter of more minor exit burns on my leg and foot. A hole in my boot completed the circuit.

As Jan was almost unscathed he drove us straight home to Edinburgh. Though beer and bed were top of my agenda we ended up in the Royal Infirmary, for a sleepless night being poked with needles and wired to ECG machines. On balance I'd have preferred the pub, but at least we gave the hard-worked medics a novel break from the usual Saturday night bottle victims. It seemed the current had missed my heart by centimetres. We'd not been fried on the spot or thrown off a cliff, and looked to have escaped post-strike …

heart failure, ruptured eardrums, internal burns and neurological damage. After a few weeks' outpatients appointments at the burns clinic my only trophy was an innocuous scar. The doctors were amazed at our good fortune. The randomness of our escape was brought home the following week when a walker was tragically killed by lightning on Ben Oss, barely 20km from The Cobbler.

Dan Bailey

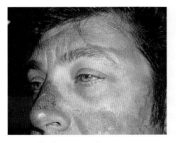

Sunburn showing superficial and partial thickness burns.
Photo: Katherine Wills

RADIATION (SUNBURN)

Caused by over exposure to the ultraviolet (UV) rays from the sun, this type of burn varies from mild redness to lobster red with blistering.

The top layer of skin may peel off a day or so after the burn, and depending on the severity there may also be pain.

WHAT TO DO

If you notice signs of the skin burning cover with clothing and move into the shade.

Cool the burn by applying cold compresses, or in the case of mild sunburn apply 'after sun' or calamine lotion.

Keep the casualty hydrated by drinking plenty of water.

Monitor this casualty for signs of dehydration, heat exhaustion and heatstroke.

TOP TIPS

Wear sun block and re-apply during the day.

Be aware that the sun reflects strongly off snow and water.

The suns rays penetrate hazy clouds therefore you can burn even on a cloudy day.

If the burn is extensive evacuate the casualty and seek further medical assistance.

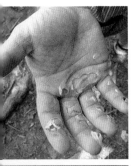

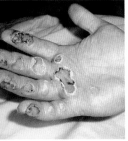

Rope burn and the same
injuries two days later.
Photos: Eric W Totel

FRICTION BURN

A burn through friction is a type of 'abrasion' caused when the skin rubs against another surface – sometimes referred to by the surface that caused the burn, for example 'rope burn'. Depending on the severity of the burn, casualties can lose several layers of skin, resulting in large open wounds which ooze clear fluid and can be very painful.

In the remote setting, friction burns are commonly seen on the backs of heels from walking boots, occasionally on hands from ropes and less frequently from a dog lead behind the legs.

WHAT TO DO

Run cold water over the burn to cool and clean it. Make sure as much dirt and debris as possible is removed from the injury.

Ideally, dead skin from torn open blisters should be carefully removed with sterilised scissors (sterilise with disinfectant or medi wipe).

Cover with a non-adherent dressing or cling film.

Monitor for infection over the next few days.

If the burn is deep or you are concerned about the injury evacuate and seek medical help.

TOP TIPS

Be very cautious with any burn to the hand. If you are unsure of the seriousness have the burn assessed at hospital.

Friction blisters on heels

It is possible to protect the feet by taping those areas prone to blistering before the start of the day. As a form of prevention some people use blister dressings instead of tape

Blisters on heels are essentially a friction burn, which is often the result of new or ill-fitting footwear. Friction causes the outer layer of skin to separate from the inner layers and the space in between fills with clear fluid (blisters caused by other means are not covered here).

Initially the casualty will be aware of the skin becoming warm and red – often referred to as a 'hot spot'. As the skin becomes more damaged, the body tries to protect itself from further rubbing and harm by producing a blister. If the blister is not protected at this stage, it can continue to rub until eventually the top is torn off, leaving an open wound.

Broken blisters

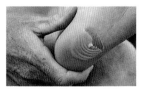

A torn blister from fell running.
Photo: Katherine Wills

Broken blisters leave the casualty with an abrasion wound, which can become embedded with dirt and bits of sock. If the skin from the top of the broken blister has clumped to one side it is recommended to remove the dead skin using sterile tweezers and scissors (sterilised with disinfectant or a medi wipe) leaving a small 2mm border of tissue around the edge. The raw skin should then be dressed using a blister plaster or equivalent.

Unbroken blisters

A small painless blister can simply be left alone and allowed to repair itself over time. Medium sized blisters can be managed with specific blister plaster. Larger blisters caused by boots or outdoor shoes can be dealt with in one of two ways; either leave the blister and try to protect it with a dressing, or drain the fluid from the blister and then dress it.

If you decide to leave the blister, attempt to protect it with a specialised blister dressing. The cushion effect of the dressing may keep the blister away from the offending footwear, stopping it bursting or tearing and thus helping to reduce discomfort.

If the blister is particularly large, or interferes with walking (or running), another option is to carefully drain the fluid, while keeping the 'roof' (top) of the blister intact. This is a common wilderness technique used widely in the remote setting when the casualty wishes to continue walking. As long as you keep the wound clean you should avoid infection.

Draining a heel blister caused by friction

- Thoroughly clean the area.

- Sterilise a needle (or safety pin) by heating it with a match until it is glowing red, then allow it to cool (alternatively sterilise with rubbing alcohol).

- Insert the sterile needle into the edge of the outer roof. Some people make a tiny 'nick' in the roof of the blister to stop it from re-sealing itself.

- Apply gentle pressure with gauze or a clean tissue to help drain the fluid.

- Cover, using a blister plaster or equivalent.

  If continuing your walk leave the roof of the blister intact as this acts as a first layer of dressing.

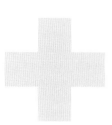

7. CARE OF WOUNDS

The term wound is used to describe any injury that damages the skin and results in a bleed. Treating wounds in a remote setting presents a number of challenges, including the lack of a sterile environment and limited first aid equipment. Wounds are either open, where the skin is damaged and the wound bleeds outwards or closed, when bleeding is contained underneath the skin (life-threatening bleeding is dealt with in a previous chapter).

Open wounds

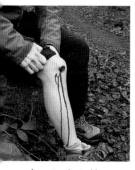

Make sure you follow your **ABC** assessment (**A**irway, **B**reathing, and **C**irculation): any airway and breathing problems must be dealt with before treating bleeding wounds.

Always take a thorough history of what exactly happened and start your treatment by putting on your examination gloves. Examine the wound carefully and in good light. Check for normal movement, blood flow and feeling beyond the wound, comparing one side of the body to the other. Clean wounds as best you can, protect by applying a suitable dressing and, if necessary, consider splinting. This approach will help to control any bleeding, minimise the chances of infection and encourage healing. If the wound is serious enough to warrant a visit to hospital, it may be useful to note the time of the accident and record if the wound was grossly contaminated.

A contaminated knee wound caused by a fall. Photo: Brian Wills

Cleaning wounds

Your ability to clean a wound in the remote setting will depend on what equipment you have available. Your options include; medi wipes, saline sachets, or drinking water. Each wound will present you with different challenges depending on its size, depth and location. Abrasions and lacerations tend to be dirty wounds and it may be necessary to remove larger bits of dirt with tweezers, and then irrigate the wound under pressure – forcefully squirting water into it.

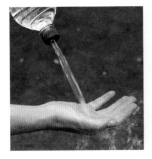

Photo: Brian Wills

IRRIGATING A WOUND

Fill a large syringe with water and then squirt it under pressure into the wound. If you don't carry a syringe, you can improvise using any of the following; a plastic bag with a small hole in the corner, a plastic water bottle with a hole punched in the lid, a CamelBak water container, or even an energy drinks bottle with a squirting top. Irrigation is not particularly painful; it doesn't do any further damage to the tissue and with sufficient pressure works really well. Use your gloved fingers to gently pry the wound open. With a grossly contaminated graze you may need to gently rub the area to help remove bits of dirt and debris. Use a piece of wet gauze, cleaning from the centre of the wound outwards. Use a clean swab each time until the wound is clean or you run out of swabs!

Children

Most children will feel somewhat frightened when they have an injury. This is particularly so in a remote setting, when the comforts of home may be a long way away. What usually appears at first sight to be a serious injury, with plenty of screams and tears, often turns out to be relatively minor and the child recovers quickly.

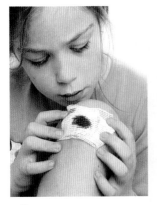

Photo:
www.istockphoto.com

TREATING CHILDREN

Ask the child exactly what happened. Allow them to tell their 'story'. Talking through their accident often makes them calm down and feel better.

Try to keep calm yourself, smile and be cheerful. If the child sees that you are stressed and anxious it will make the situation worse.

If the child is young and a parent is present (and the injury allows), let the child sit on the parent's lap during the treatment. If possible try to demonstrate any treatments on the parent first, so they can see what is going to happen.

Avoid standing over the child; sit or kneel next to them as you talk.

Explain everything you are doing, using words they can understand.

If the child is young, try to distract them with toys or games.

Different types of open wounds

Open wounds include; incised (cut), abrasion (graze), laceration (jagged tear), puncture (hole), embedded object (something sticking out), gunshot, skin loss and skin flap. It is possible your casualty will present you with more than one type of wound. A common sense approach is needed when managing wounds in the remote setting; most casualties will simply require some basic first aid treatment then sent on their way. However on occasions wounds may be so severe they will need an emergency response and immediate evacuation.

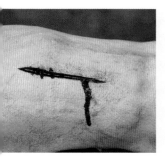

INCISED WOUND

An incised wound is caused by a sharp-edged object; such as a knife, slate, etc. The severity of the wound will depend on its location and depth. Incised wounds have the potential to cut through ligaments, tendons and nerves deeper in the body and in severe cases may pierce major blood vessels – resulting in a potentially life-threatening bleed.

WHAT TO DO

Examine the wound carefully to make sure the sharp object that caused the injury is not embedded.

Clean the wound.

Consider wound closure strips or if not suitable apply a dressing according to the amount of leakage.

If necessary elevate the wound above the heart and consider splinting.

TOP TIPS

Never stitch wounds with a needle and thread, or glue them closed.

If bleeding is significant, apply direct pressure quickly, using your gloved hand, or improvise.

Elevate the limb at the same time. Maintain the pressure for at least 10 minutes. Avoid the temptation to keep looking as this can restart bleeding.

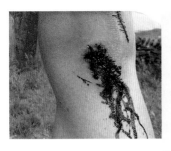

Abrasion.
Photo: Kate Worthington

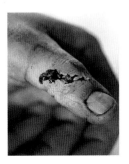

Laceration.
Photo:
www.istockphoto.com

ABRASION (GRAZE) AND LACERATION

Abrasions are a relatively superficial wound to the top layer of the skin, usually from a sliding fall onto a hard surface. They often contain dirt, gravel or other debris, and 'ooze' blood. They can be quite painful, difficult to clean and are prone to infection.

A laceration is a rough, jagged tear-like wound. The depth of the damage to the skin can vary depending on the mechanisms of injury. Your treatment will depend on the depth of the wound.

Deep lacerations can damage not only blood vessels, but also tendons and nerves. These wounds can be contaminated with dirt, gravel and other debris, similar to an abrasion.

WHAT TO DO

Carefully examine the wound.

Clean, using pressure irrigation – you may not be able to remove all foreign material, but try to clean the larger bits. Avoid sending dirt and debris from the undamaged skin into the wound itself.

Cover with a dressing according to the size and amount of bleeding. It may be necessary to apply another bulky dressing over the top to absorb any discharge and protect from further damage.

TOP TIPS

If you are unable to remove all the bits of dirt and debris during cleaning, you will have to re-clean once you are out of the remote setting. For grossly contaminated wounds self-evacuate then take to hospital.

It is important to monitor these wounds for infection.

For deep lacerations on an extremity (arm or leg) consider splinting; this helps keep the dressing in place.

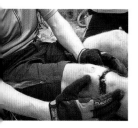

REAL
LIFE
STORY

Colin's injury.
Photos: Sabine Hoekema

Laceration

A bend hid most of the big rock section near the end but I knew it was there. I chose my line and slowed down. Unfortunately a rock moved under my front wheel and snatched my bars sideways. As I was thrown forwards my rear wheel left the ground. This gave me two choices, face-plant into rocks or bail to the side for a soft landing on grass. No contest, the grass won.

By the time I hit, I'd lost most of my speed and can't have been doing more than 5mph. Unfortunately my knee struck the edge of the top bolt of my brake lever bar when I landed. It penetrated the skin just below my kneecap and didn't come out; my knee tore, like opening a crisp packet.

When I rolled out of the accident and looked down, I couldn't believe what I saw. There was an 8-inch horizontal tear in my knee! I grabbed the skin above and below the wound to hold it together.

"Can you get my first aid kit?" I asked "It's in my back pack". There was no way I was letting go of my leg to hunt for it myself. Before I knew it Anne, Ed and Brian had sprung into action. Stupidly I hadn't replenished my stock of steri-strips, but Ed said he had some. While he retrieved his first aid kit, I realised that the huge hole in my leg wasn't bleeding and there was no pain.

"Put this on", "It's not big enough", "I can stick a few together", "Okay". "I've found this as well", "But that's not big enough either!", "Yes, but I've opened it! Stick it on anyway", "Okay". Something else was opened and handed to Ed "That's a bloody eye patch, what am I going to do with that?"

With the first aid underway, I was free to sort out my evacuation. I showed Tom where we were on the map, and the nearest place with communication, before he went with half the group to get help.

It would be easier for the emergency services to recover me from the road, rather than 200m up a very rocky track. I was sure I could make it down without causing further damage. With my knee quickly covered, I dropped the saddle and slowly free-wheeled down.

At the A&E in Sheffield, I was soon attended by a doctor. "So how did you do this?" he asked. I told him. "So how's your bike?" came the reply. Fantastic, he was a mountain biker. After inspecting my wound he called his mate over. "Guess how he did this". The second doctor was told, and he asked, "So how's your bike?" Cool, two mountain biking doctors.
                                                                    ...

Giving first aid.

My wound was too big for A&E, so I was sent up to surgery. After the operation, I got the results. It was good news. It had taken 18 stitches to sew up my leg but there was no structural damage, and I could be back on a bike within 2–4 weeks. You dont know how relieved I was.

Colin Down

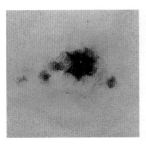

Photo: Brian Wills

PUNCTURE WOUND

Puncture wounds are caused by something piercing the skin, creating a hole. This can be superficial, only involving the surface of the skin, or deep, including ligaments, tendons, nerves, large blood vessels and/or internal organs.

The external wound itself does not usually bleed significantly (unless it has pierced a large blood vessel), but the risk of infection is high. If the object is still in the wound, leave it in place and treat as for an embedded object.

WHAT TO DO

Carefully examine the wound.

Allow the wound to bleed; this will help wash out dirt and bacteria.

Clean the wound.

Cover with a dressing and secure in place.

TOP TIPS

The problem with this type of wound is infection, caused by debris and bacteria entering the tissue.

Deep puncture wounds to the chest or abdomen can also pierce underlying vital organs and can be serious. This is an emergency.

Dial 999/112 – request police – then ask for mountain rescue.

Insulate from the ground, provide shelter and monitor vital signs: level of response (AVPU), breathing and pulse, while you await rescue.

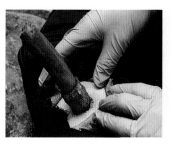

EMBEDDED OBJECT

Do not remove any object that is embedded in the casualty.
Unnecessary removal of these objects may cause further damage.
For example, wood may leave splinters behind. The embedded object may also be pushing against a main blood vessel creating a 'plug' and reducing blood loss; removal could create a significant bleed.

WHAT TO DO

Check the wound carefully.

Do not attempt to move or remove the object, if necessary cut away clothing to expose the embedded object and skin.

Apply pressure around the edges of the wound and the object using either your hands or the casualty's. Do not apply pressure on top of the embedded object itself.

Replace this pressure with dressings and padding and secure in place; this stops the embedded object from moving.

Large embedded objects – it may be necessary for you to support the object with your hands, or secure it in place with more bulky items of padding.

If the object is large or deeply embedded, you will need assistance.

Dial 999/112 – request police – then ask for mountain rescue.

Insulate from the ground, provide shelter and monitor the vital signs: level of response (AVPU), breathing and pulse, while you await rescue.

TOP TIP

If the casualty is impaled (they are stuck on an object as opposed to the object being stuck into them) support their body to stop any unnecessary movement which could cause further damage.

Dial 999/112 – request police – then ask for mountain rescue.

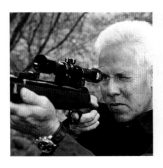

GUNSHOT WOUND

This wound is actually an 'unpredictable' puncture wound and can involve major tissue damage, including splintered or shattered bones and damage to vital organs. The seriousness of this wound will depend on where the casualty has been shot, the size of the bullet, the speed it was travelling and the distance of the gun from the casualty.

WHAT TO DO

Dial 999/112 – request police – then ask for mountain rescue.

Remember **danger** is your first consideration. Any situation that involves a gun has the potential to be hazardous.

Follow your **ABC** approach – if the casualty is unconscious deal with them accordingly, if not breathing start basic life support (CPR).

Control any bleeding.

If the injury is to the chest, cover the wound with something airtight and seal around three sides.

Conscious casualties will find the most comfortable position for themselves. Unconscious casualties must be placed into a **safe airway position**.

Insulate from the ground, provide shelter and monitor the casualty's vital signs: level of response (AVPU), breathing and pulse, while you await rescue.

TOP TIPS

Gunshot wounds may create both entrance and exit wounds. It is not always possible to work out which is which, so don't! Simply identify them as wounds and treat accordingly.

Anyone who has suffered a gunshot wound should be seen in hospital immediately, regardless of how minor the injury appears.

If after applying an airtight dressing on a chest wound the casualty starts to deteriorate remove it immediately (see chapter on **Breathing Problems**).

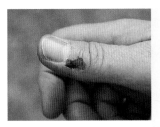

Skinl loss.
Photo: Brian Wills

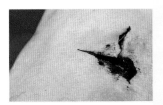

Skin flap.

SKIN LOSS AND SKIN FLAPS

Skin loss wounds are caused by forces that run parallel to the skin, which forcibly tear or 'shave' the skin away. These wounds can be:

Minor – a small area involving only the surface skin layers.

Moderate – a significant amount of skin is removed and may include deeper tissue.

Severe – in cases of near or complete amputation.

Skin flaps are similar to skin loss; however the skin is not torn completely off, but creates a flap. These can vary from superficial, involving only the surface of the skin, to deep, including fat and muscle.

Small skin flaps often heal with few complications or infection. Deep skin flaps, involving fat and muscle tissue, require evacuation because they tend to heal poorly and become infected easily.

WHAT TO DO

Check and clean the wound carefully.

Treat the injury.

Skin loss – Cover with a non adherent dressing and secure in place. It may be necessary to apply another bulky dressing over the top to absorb any discharge and protect from further damage.

Skin flap – Remove any dirt from the wound and then replace the flap of skin over the wound and secure it in place with a bulky dressing soaked in saline to keep the flap moist.

TOP TIPS

Deep skin loss wounds on an extremity, for example an arm or leg, can be dressed and then splinted.

Large skin loss and skin flap wounds that include fat and muscle can be quite incapacitating. Therefore you may have to seek outside help.

...

Dial 999/112 – request police – then ask for mountain rescue.

Insulate from the ground, provide shelter and monitor vital signs: level of response (AVPU), breathing and pulse, while you await rescue.

Closed wounds (bruise)

Bruises are common and involve damage to the tiny blood vessels under the skin, causing a thin layer of blood to fan out from the injury. Damage to larger blood vessels deeper in the tissue can create a more significant bleed causing the area to swell; this is a kind of deep lumpy bruise (hematoma) and can be quite painful.

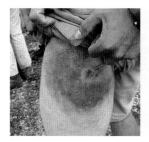

Photo: David French

BRUISE

Bruises are actually a crush injury, which damages tissue and causes bleeding under the skin. The vast majority of bruises are relatively minor and do not cause any concerns. On occasions however they can be huge, particularly if on the thigh or buttock, and for some be quite disabling.

WHAT TO DO

Bruises sometimes overlie fractured bones; check thoroughly.

If available immerse the body part in cold water (such as a mountain stream), or cover with wet towels or clothing. If ice or snow is available, these can be applied after the skin has been covered.

Elevate the body part above the heart to help reduce swelling.

TOP TIPS

This wound requires rest and the application of a cold pack, which in the remote setting may be impossible!

Never place ice or snow directly onto skin.

A few hours after a severe bruise on the thigh or hip, the limb may become so stiff and sore that the casualty may be unable to walk: you may need to re-assess your planned journey.

Special wounds

This section includes wounds to the hands, feet and amputations. Injuries to the ears, eyes, nose and mouth are dealt with in detail in the chapter on **Head, Scalp, Face and Eye Injuries**.

Hands and feet

Wounds to the hands and feet must be dealt with cautiously; all but the most superficial injuries are treated as serious. Apart from obvious wounds to the skin, injuries to tendons, ligaments, nerves or blood vessels can cause severe and disabling impairment. Always check sensation and circulation beyond the injury.

When bandaging fingers or toes it is sometimes useful to place gauze, or some other protective dressing, between the digits in order to prevent damage to the skin from dampness created by sweating, particularly if the casualty is to spend some time in the remote setting.

Amputation

Traumatic amputations in the remote setting are not as uncommon as you might think.

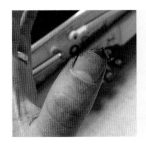

Photo: Fiona Moore

AMPUTATION

Parts of the body that have been cut or torn off are said to be amputated, either partially or completely. It is possible to re-attach some amputated parts therefore you should make every effort to retrieve it/them. Complications include blood loss shock (depending on the location and nature of the injury) and infection.

WHAT TO DO

Follow your **ABC** approach.

Try to calm the casualty, as an amputation can be frightening.

Check the wound carefully.

Control bleeding and dress accordingly.

If the amputation causes significant blood loss treat for shock.   ...

Complete amputation – If the amputated part can be found note the time of the amputation.

If small, rinse in clean water to remove dirt and wrap in gauze or anything clean. Place in a plastic bag, (examination glove if small enough), or waterproof container. If available place this container in ice or snow. **Never** place the amputated part directly **in** water.

Partial amputation – If medical help is some time away return the limb to its normal position and immobilise the part with bulky dressings.

Splint the limb to prevent any further injury.

Dial 999/112 – request police – then ask for mountain rescue.

Insulate from the ground, provide shelter and monitor vital signs: level of response (AVPU), breathing and pulse, while awaiting rescue.

REAL
LIFE
STORY

Finger amputation

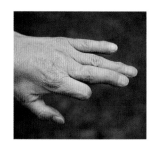

I was belaying at the foot of a sea crag when a sudden shout made me look up. A large rock was hurtling towards me. I ducked to one side. Then came an explosion of sound and I saw stars. As the dust settled, I felt the weight of my partner on the rope and I assumed the worst. 'Are you OK?' I yelled. 'Yes' came the reply, 'how about you?'

Seeing stars made me think I'd been hit on the head, but as I scanned my body I could feel no pain. I looked down at my torso and legs and along my right arm to my hand; all fine. I began to relax and was about to tell my partner that I was OK, when I looked across to my left hand. What a mess! Middle finger and thumb hanging off and index finger completely severed.

I lowered my partner down and he took off his T-shirt, bound my hand, got me to elevate it, checked me for other injuries and climbed out for help. On reaching the top of the cliff he found some people to help haul me up. He gave my finger to some others, who put it in a cool bag and got some ice from the local pub to keep it cool. The coastguard had arrived by this time. They were very keen to check my hand, but I didn't want them near it. Nothing useful could be done until I got to hospital, and I knew I couldn't deal with seeing it again, or with their reaction.

There was no pain as such. Instead I felt uncomfortable and agitated. Like the feeling of desperately needing the loo!   …

When I got into the helicopter I couldn't see the bag that contained my finger and panicked until the winch-man put it next to me on the seat. As we approached the hospital, the pain increased and I was worried about how long it would take to be seen by a doctor. Fortunately, it wasn't long before I was breathing in gas and air and giggling happily.

It took three operations and eleven months to sort out my thumb and middle finger. Despite the fact that the index finger arrived in perfect condition, I didn't have it sewn back on. If I had, I was told, I would not have been able to bend it and climbing would have been a problem. However, knowing I had it with me was psychologically very important.

Eluned Roberts

Complications

Bleeding and clotting

It is useful during your treatment to ask the casualty if they have any medical conditions or are taking any medication. It is particularly important to establish if they have a bleeding disorder, such as haemophilia, which affects the body's ability to clot blood. A bleeding casualty with a known blood disorder, or those taking medications to thin the blood (such as warfarin), can experience heavy and prolonged bleeding.

Wound infection

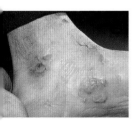

Photo: Bryn Williams

All open wounds in the remote setting are considered to be contaminated and as such have the potential to become infected. If the casualty is to spend several days in the remote environment, it may be sensible to inspect the wound every day for signs of infection, and change the dressing every 24 to 48 hours. If you are in a particularly hot and sweaty environment, or the dressing becomes wet or dirty, you may need to change it more regularly. If you detect signs of infection, it would be wise to self-evacuate the casualty and seek medical assistance.

INFECTED WOUNDS

The following are signs of infection:

Tissue around the wound swells.   …

Redness spreading out from the wound.

If the wound is open, you may see pus leaking. It may be thick and creamy yellow or white, or watery with a light green colour.

The wound feels warm to touch.

Increasing pain and tenderness.

The casualty develops a fever.

Swollen glands.

Generally feeling unwell – nausea, poor appetite.

Tetanus

Tetanus (lockjaw), is a serious bacterial infection which causes muscle spasms and stiffness throughout the body (particularly in the neck, face and jaw), and can be fatal.

The bacteria are usually found in soil, dust and manure and normally enter the body through an open wound on the skin. Due to the vaccination programme started in 1961 tetanus infection in the UK is quite rare. However if the wound is contaminated with dirt which is prone to tetanus, for example manure, an immunoglobulin injection will be required; therefore the casualty should be seen at hospital.

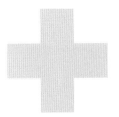

8. FRACTURES, DISLOCATIONS AND SPRAINS

These types of injuries usually require a common sense approach: not all will need an emergency response. You may be able to deal with the injury yourself and with a little physical and emotional support evacuate the casualty without assistance. However, sometimes they can be extremely painful and incapacitating, on occasions creating serious limb-threatening and even life-threatening problems. You will need to develop an understanding of those injuries that can be managed and those that require urgent evacuation.

The skeleton

The skeleton gives us our human shape providing a bony rigid support. When two or more bones meet they create a joint and these are supported by ligaments (tough leathery tissue), which connect bones to each other. Muscles are the pulley system which create movement and are connected to bones via tendons. Despite being strong, bones can break (fracture), joints can become displaced (dislocation), ligaments can stretch and tear (sprains) and muscles and tendons can overstretch (strains).

Fractures

Fractures are referred to as being either **open** or **closed**. Open fractures involve some kind of wound on the skin over the broken bone and on occasions the bone may be sticking through the skin. These types of fractures carry a very high risk of infection. In closed fractures the skin above the break is intact. It is not important to know the medical names of bones; keep it simple and refer to them by their commonly used terms – such as collar bone, upper arm, etc.

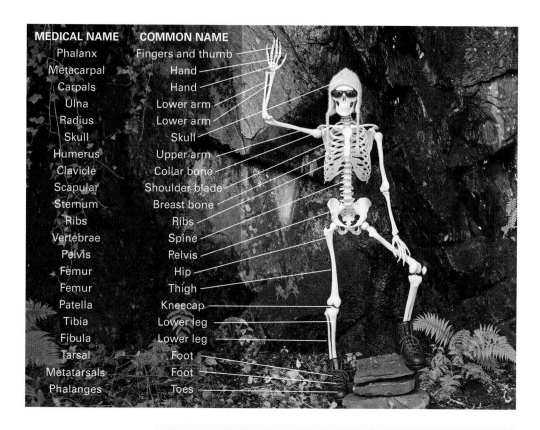

MEDICAL NAME	COMMON NAME
Phalanx	Fingers and thumb
Metacarpal	Hand
Carpals	Hand
Ulna	Lower arm
Radius	Lower arm
Skull	Skull
Humerus	Upper arm
Clavicle	Collar bone
Scapular	Shoulder-blade
Sternum	Breast bone
Ribs	Ribs
Vertebrae	Spine
Pelvis	Pelvis
Femur	Hip
Femur	Thigh
Patella	Kneecap
Tibia	Lower leg
Fibula	Lower leg
Tarsal	Foot
Metatarsals	Foot
Phalanges	Toes

Part of your initial assessment should be to establish the mechanisms of injury; ask the casualty or witnesses "what happened?" Understanding the forces involved will help guide you to suspect certain types of injuries.

HOW WE BREAK BONES

High energy – Accidents involving extreme forces can damage bones, soft tissue and internal organs. Any fall from over-head height is considered high energy.

Direct blow – The fracture occurs at the point of impact.

Twisting – This is common in the remote setting.

Indirect force – Falls can cause injury further up the limb than the point of contact.

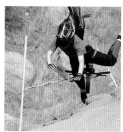
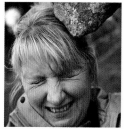
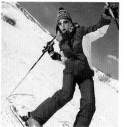
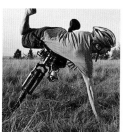

Photo: www.istockphoto.com   Photo: www.istockphoto.com Photo: www.istockphoto.com

Potential life-threatening fractures

Bones rarely break in isolation; there is usually some damage to muscles, tendons, ligaments or blood vessels nearby. Blood loss can be a huge problem, particularly with a broken thigh bone or pelvis; breaks to just one of these bones may cause your casualty to go into shock and can be life-threatening. In fact any fracture that causes a problem in your primary survey – **ABC** assessment – is serious and requires urgent evacuation.

Airway problems:

- Skull fractures: unconscious, unable to maintain their airway.

- Some facial fractures.

Breathing problems:

- Rib fractures and flail chest injuries.

- High spinal fractures.

Circulation problems:

- Open fractures with significant external bleeding.

- Thigh bone fracture.

- Pelvic fracture.

- Rib fractures that puncture organs causing internal bleeding.

Identifying a fracture

It is difficult to tell the difference between a broken bone and a severe injury to muscle, tendon or ligaments – unless of course the bone is obviously deformed. However there are a number of signs and symptoms that will guide you to suspect a fracture, although these may vary from individual to individual and injury to injury. In all honesty it doesn't really matter because you treat what you find. If the casualty falls, says their leg hurts and they can't walk on it, treat as if it is broken.

This photograph shows what is meant by 'skin tenting': when the deformity of the bone underneath stretches the skin, which turns white. This is serious.
Photo: Paul Smith

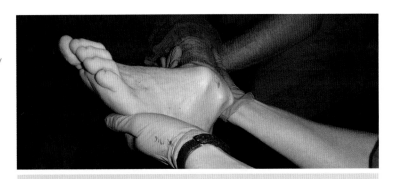

LOOK OUT FOR

Immediate pain – made worse when the limb is moved.

Rapid swelling.

Bruising – some time later.

Loss of function – unable to use the limb.

Deformity – appears misshapen and if grossly deformed skin tenting (skin stretching over a damaged bone).

An open wound at the break, sometimes with the bone sticking out.

Crepitus – grinding or cracking noise.

Assessing and controlling pain

Pain is unpleasant and every attempt should be made to reduce distress and discomfort. This starts early with your ability to put the casualty at ease – don't underestimate the effects of a reassuring and confident approach.

To gauge how much pain a casualty is feeling, you can use a **pain score scale**, ranging from zero to ten.

PAIN SCORE SCALE

Ask the casualty something like: "On a scale of 0 to 10, with 0 being no pain and 10 being the worst pain imaginable, what score would you give the pain you feel if your fracture is moved a little?"

0	1	2	3	4	5	6	7	8	9	10

no pain   mild pain   moderate pain   severe pain   worst pain ever

The simplest way of controlling fracture (and dislocation) pain, is to stop the fracture or joint from moving; splint by immobilising the joint above and below the injury. For a deformed lower limb fracture, there is the additional option of applying manual traction (pulling the broken limb back into line with your hands) if medical help is some time away, and you are trained and feel confident to do so. In an urban setting it is inappropriate to realign broken limbs if an ambulance is only minutes away. In the remote environment however, when help may take some considerable time, applying traction can result in less long-term damage to the limb.

For issues surrounding carrying and offering medication, see the chapter Outdoor First Aid Kits.

You may be in a position to offer over-the-counter oral painkillers such as paracetamol, ibubrofen, co-codamol (paracetamol plus codeine), co-dydramol (paracetamol plus dihydrocodeine) or ibubrofen plus codeine. If calling for the rescue services it is important that any medication taken by the casualty is written down – including the name of the drug, dose and time – and handed to them on their arrival.

Splinting

Before moving a casualty, all broken bones and dislocations should be splinted, unless in grave danger when the priority should be to urgently move the casualty to safety. Splinting stops the injury from moving and can reduce pain and swelling, help to avoid further damage to muscle and other soft tissue, and potentially prevent a closed fracture becoming open. Splints can also be used to secure dressings in place, helping to control bleeding.

WHAT TO DO

To be effective a splint needs to completely stop all movement at the site of the injury and the joints above and below.

If possible remove clothing, rings and watches from the area and examine the injury carefully.

Dress all wounds.

Check circulation and sensation beyond the site of the injury.

Place padding between the splint and the skin to prevent pressure and discomfort.

If using a splint secure it to the body with ties or a bandage.

Recheck circulation and sensation beyond the site of the injury after splinting is complete.

The easiest way of splinting is to use the casualty's own body (if possible); for example taping a fractured finger to the adjacent one. There are very versatile commercially produced splints such as the SAM Splint – or you may be able to improvise with what ever equipment is to hand.

A popular shop-bought splint used in the outdoors is the SAM Splint, which is a flexible, lightweight, soft metal sheet padded on both sides with foam.

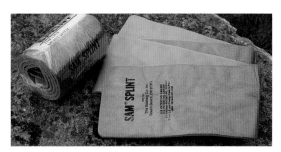

Improvised Splints

Splints can be improvised from many things, such as Karrimats (used for camping), the stiff foam pad at the back of a rucksack, tent poles fanned out, taped and padded, or even walking poles. Basically any stiffened object that stops the limb from moving about can be used as a splint. It is important to use plenty of **padding**; improvise with spare fleeces, hats, gloves, etc.

TENT OR WALKING POLES: BROKEN LOWER ARM

The poles are taped together and padding placed between the injured arm and the splint.

Secure the splint in place with a bandage or ties, leaving a gap at the wrist to check for a pulse.

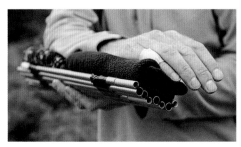
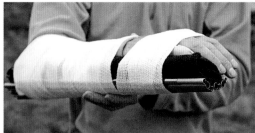

KARRIMAT: BROKEN LOWER LEG

Lay your mat beside leg. Extend mat the same length as the casualty's foot past the heal. Fold the top part over so the top edge sits level with the crotch. Place padding level with the knee and lower leg including the foot. Keep padding flat and unwrinkled.   ...

*Remember to get all your equipment together and ready – splint, padding, ties or bandages to secure the splint – **before** you move the injured limb!*

Support lower leg and slid the mat underneath. Position ties by sliding up underneath the mat. Avoid unnecessary movement of the injured leg. If available place two ties above and one below the kneecap, and one at the ankle. Avoid placing ties over the kneecap or injury.

Bring the sides of the mat together to compress and secure in place with your ties. Keep ties wide where they lie over skin or alternatively pad underneath. Tie with a bow to allow adjustment.

At the foot take all the padding and mat beyond the foot and fold up to create a T-shape. Bring the wings of the T around and fold them inwards encircling the foot. Use your final tie to secure around the base of the foot and wings. Again tie with a bow to allow for adjustment.

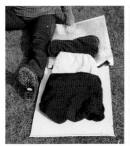 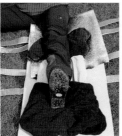 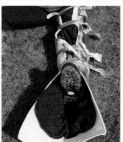 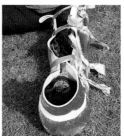

Children and fractures

Most broken bones in children occur in the upper limbs, particularly the wrist, forearm and around the elbow. Their bones are different from those of adults; they tend to be more pliable and bend further without breaking.

Treating fractures

Here are some principles to consider when treating a possible fracture.

WHAT TO DO

Take a history of exactly what happened.

Follow your **ABC**s.

Examine the fracture using the 'Look, Feel, Move' approach:

Look: for wounds, swelling and deformity.   ...

Feel: for tenderness, any loss of feeling.

Move: can the casualty move or weight bear on the limb? Don't ask them to move an obvious fracture!

Assess their level of pain and consider offering pain relief.

Remove all jewellery from the injured area if possible, including rings, watches and bracelets.

If appropriate clean any fracture wounds. Dress all wounds.

Limb fractures: check circulation and sensation below the suspected fracture site **before** and **after** splinting.

Deformed lower leg fractures: apply manual traction – if medical help is some time away and you are trained and confident to do so.

Splint the limb.

If the fracture is not serious, consider self-evacuation, otherwise:

Dial 999/112 – request police – then ask for mountain rescue.

Insulate from the ground, provide shelter, re-assess their level of pain and monitor your casualty while you await rescue.

The 'Look, Feel, Move' method of assessing a fracture is great in principle, but sometimes in the remote setting it is incredibly difficult. What is important is that you attempt to establish the likelihood of a fracture, endeavour to dress any wounds and stop the fracture from moving about by immobilising, for instance splint.

If there is an open wound over the fracture site, the current advice is to **only** clean it if there is gross contamination – such as lumps of grass or manure. Otherwise simply cover with a dressing and evacuate to hospital.

Fractures – specific locations

This section deals with fractures of the collar bone, arm, hand, fingers and thumbs, pelvis, thigh, lower leg and ankle. Rib fractures are discussed in the chapter **Breathing Problems**; skull fractures and fractures of the face in the chapter **Head, Scalp, Face and Eye Injuries** and injuries to the spine in the chapter **Spine and Back Injuries**.

Remember, don't become distracted by an obvious fracture – always follow your **ABC**s. When dealing with a broken bone in a casualty who is fit, young and healthy take the time to consider carefully the forces involved; you will need to check for other potential injuries.

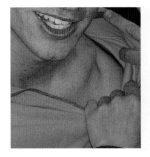

Photo: Steven Smith

COLLAR-BONE FRACTURE

These fractures can happen from a fall onto the shoulder, a direct blow to the collar bone, or through indirect forces from a fall onto an outstretched hand. On occasions you may notice an obvious step in the bone, with the skin looking like its being stretched (tenting). The arm on the injured side is usually bent at the elbow and held across the chest, with the other arm supporting it.

WHAT TO DO

Immobilise the arm on the injured side.

Evacuate the casualty and take to hospital.

TOP TIPS

The collar bone sits at the top of the chest. Be mindful of this and check for any possible underlying chest injury, as well as head or neck injuries.

A fractured collar bone is **serious** if: the fracture is open, there is obvious stretching of the skin over the fracture site (tenting), or if there are other significant injuries to the chest.

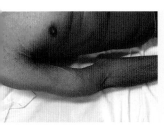

UPPER ARM

These fractures can occur from a direct blow to the upper arm, or indirectly from a fall onto an outstretched arm. They may on occasions include nerve damage with a loss or a change of sensation in the lower arm.

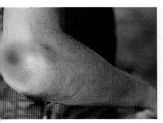

ELBOW

Elbow fractures are common in children and usually happen with a fall onto the outstretched hand. Fractured elbows in adults tend to occur as a result of a direct blow to the elbow. The casualty is unable to bend or stretch out the elbow.

Photo: Amber Schoessow

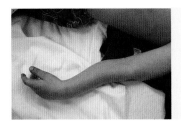

FOREARM

There are two bones in the forearm. They can break close to the elbow, in the middle or at the wrist. These injuries can happen from a fall onto the outstretched hand or from a direct blow to the forearm.

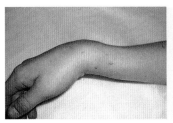

WRIST

Wrist injuries usually occur from a fall onto the outstretched hand or from a direct blow to the wrist. If deformed, the wrist often bends like a 'dinner fork'. If the casualty falls onto the back of the arm, the wrist bends the other way.

Photo: www.ski-injury.com

WHAT TO DO

Check circulation at the wrist and sensation in the fingers.

Immobilise the arm in a position that is most comfortable.

Upper arm – If possible gently place the forearm horizontally across the chest and immobilise with an arm sling.

To add support secure the arm to the chest by applying a broad bandage (avoid securing it over the fracture site).

Elbow – Immobilise with an arm sling, or use broad bandages and plenty of padding to secure to the body.

Forearm and wrist – If available apply a splint or improvise. If not, use plenty of padding and immobilise the arm using an arm sling.

To add support, secure the arm to the chest with a broad bandage.

All of the above – Re-check circulation and sensation at the wrist.

If not serious, consider self-evacuation then take to hospital.

Treat as an **Emergency** if:

Pain is severe (pain score of between 7 and 10).

The fracture is grossly deformed.

Reduced or no circulation at the wrist.   ...

Change of sensation down the arm or hand.

Open fracture.

Other injuries, or you are some distance from your transport.

Dial 999/112 – request police – then ask for mountain rescue.

Insulate from the ground, provide shelter and monitor your casualty while you await rescue.

TOP TIPS

Be extremely cautious with children who have any injury around the elbow that causes pain, swelling or bruising, or if they are unable to bend and straighten the elbow properly.

In forearm fractures where both bones are broken, there is a risk that the bone ends will break through the skin (open fracture). It is important to immobilise the arm to stop this happening.

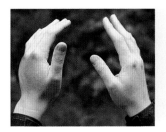

HAND, FINGER AND THUMB FRACTURES

Hand fractures can happen in either the small bones of the fingers and thumb, or the longer bones that form the back of the hand and palm. These fractures commonly occur as a result of a direct fall or blow to the hand, as well as a crush injury.

WHAT TO DO

Finger and thumb injury – Thinly pad between the fingers and lightly strap the injury to its neighbour using tape.

Swelling will occur, therefore monitor this injury; you may need to loosen the tape.

For both fingers and thumb injuries, place in an elevated sling to help control pain and reduce swelling.

Hand injury – Immobilise the hand and place in an elevated sling, using plenty of padding.

Evacuate, and then take to hospital.

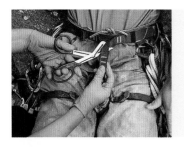

PELVIC FRACTURES

The concern with this injury is the potential for the bone ends to cut through major blood vessels that lie on the inside of the pelvis, causing life-threatening internal bleeding. The casualty complains of pain and tenderness in the pelvis. If the fracture has severed a large blood vessel the casualty will go into shock.

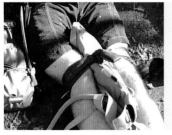

THIGH FRACTURES

The casualty is normally in severe pain and will be unable to walk. There is obvious swelling at the site of the injury and some degree of deformity; the leg may be shortened or sticking out at a strange angle. It's not uncommon for these fractures to be open and bleeding. This injury will cause the casualty to go into shock.

Photos: Steve Gough

WHAT TO DO

Urgently dial 999/112, request police, then ask for mountain rescue.

Follow your **ABC** approach.

Treat the injury:

Pelvic injury – do not touch the pelvis. Your assessment should **only** involve establishing the mechanisms of injury (what happened!) and if conscious, the casualty's symptoms.

Within the UK remote setting the first aid guidance is to do very little with this injury. If possible bring the knees together, pad in between, then immobilise the legs by tying them together. If movement causes increased pain then stop and simply surround the area with soft padding (such as spare clothing).

Thigh bone – If this is an open fracture external bleeding should be controlled.

Check circulation and sensation at the ankle.

If the casualty will allow (and you feel confident about doing this) the advice from orthopedic and emergency medicine specialists working in UK mountain rescue suggest grasping the ankle of the injured leg and applying gentle continuous manual traction.   ...

Secure the injured leg to the good one using plenty of padding between the knees and ankles.

Re-check circulation and sensation at the ankle.

Treat for blood loss shock.

If possible insulate from the ground, provide shelter and monitor vital signs: level of response (AVPU), breathing and pulse, while you await rescue.

TOP TIPS

These injuries are an **emergency**. It is likely that casualties with these types of fractures also have other significant injuries (including internal), as well as a possible spinal injury.

Do not move these casualties unless they are in danger or they have an airway problem you need to sort out.

Shock is a significant feature with these injuries.

Do not log roll the pelvic fracture casualty.

Broken thigh bones need a specialist traction splint. There are a number of 'improvised' techniques out there, however due to the normally relatively short rescue time within the UK remote setting, it is generally advised to await specialist equipment from a rescue team, rather than creating a 'make do' device.

LOWER LEG AND ANKLE FRACTURES

Lower leg – Fractures of the shin bones can occur from a direct blow, or a twisting motion when the foot is fixed (i.e. between two rocks or when skiing) and the upper body rotates around it. Between the shin bone and the injury there is very little tissue, therefore these fractures may be open.

Deformity is common and usually obvious – sometimes causing the lower half of the leg to stick out at a weird angle.

Ankle – Ankle fractures usually happen due to rotation of the foot, or occasionally through a direct blow.   ...

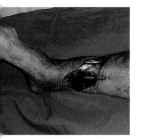

Photo: Glynne Andrew

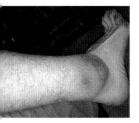

Photo: Gruff Owen

Most ankle injuries turn out to be sprains of the ligaments on the outside, caused by the foot turning inward, but it is difficult to tell the difference between a nasty sprain and a fracture. Ligament injuries and fractures often happen together and on occasions the ankle can be dislocated as well.

If in doubt assume a fracture and treat accordingly.

WHAT TO DO

Check circulation and sensation below the site of the injury.

Treat the injury:

Lower leg – Dress all wounds.

Immobilise by splinting.

Deformed lower leg – Realigning the lower leg and ankle (manual traction) if you are trained and feel confident to do so.

Ideally, any deformity in the shin bone should be corrected by manual traction at the ankle (gently pulling), as early as possible. It may be necessary for another person to hold above the fracture site to provide a stable base from which to pull. Once pulling, if the foot is rotated return it back to its original position then, whilst continuing to pull, return the leg back to its normal position, side by side with the uninjured leg. Maintain traction until the leg is immobilised.

You must be confident about what you are doing; if you are unsure leave the leg alone and call for assistance.

Ankle – Splint ankle and foot injuries using a splint or improvise. If possible avoid tying this injury to the other leg, use a separate splint.

Re-check circulation and sensation below the site of the injury.

If necessary:

Dial 999/112 – request police – then ask for mountain rescue.

Insulate from the ground, provide shelter and monitor your casualty whilst you await rescue.

TOP TIPS

Fractures of the lower leg and ankle are the most common injury dealt with by mountain rescue teams in the UK.

If applying manual traction, make a note on your **casualty report form** if circulation and sensation improved after straightening and immobilisation. If after applying traction and returning the limb to its normal position you find that circulation and sensation are actually worse, move it back to its deformed position and leave it there. Inform the rescue team on their arrival.

REAL LIFE STORY

Broken lower leg

I was facing outward, crouching slightly and slowly walking toward the apex of the convex slab of rock. Suddenly I was unbalanced, I was moving quicker, I was airborne. My gaze was fixed on the small but harmful looking boulders where I knew my journey was to terminate abruptly.

My left foot landed firmly in between two small boulders, the weight and momentum of my upper body and rucksack wrenched on my leg. There was a loud sharp snap like dry wood being broken for a fire. I was aware of the loud, shrill cries of pain emanating from my mouth. I looked down to see a right angled bend about halfway between my knee and my ankle, and a sharp point of bone trying to make its way out of my trouser leg.

I held the swaying ankle and slowly put it back into position, the grating of bone on bone was agonising. I grasped my ankle and groveled my way from the boulders to a clear, sloping area of leaves and mud. Between pants, screams of pain and floods of tears, I urged Travis my friend to take his time.

When he got to me, I was cradling my pathetically limp foot in my arms. He looked at my face, then at my leg, then at my face again; he looked like he was going to vomit. I told him we needed to splint it. He produced some weak looking twigs, I looked doubtful, his eyes lit up and he removed the two metal strips from his rucksacks back support. My long sleeve thermal was then wound round my leg and the improvised splints applied.

Travis then left to get help and the passage of time was hazy and immeasurable. It was several hours before I heard the reassuring thudding of a helicopter in-bound. Help was here at last.

Trystan Jones-Morris

Dislocations

Dislocations happen when joints move out of their normal place. As a general rule dislocations should only be put back in (reduced) by those medically trained to do so; attempting to reduce a joint without appropriate instruction may result in a significantly worse injury.

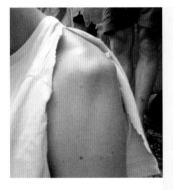

Photo: Steve Howe

Photo: Tracy Diggle

SHOULDER AND ELBOW DISLOCATIONS

Shoulder dislocation – The shoulder joint has an amazing range of movement and as a result is vulnerable to dislocating. It can be extremely painful, and the casualty often holds and supports the arm on the injured side in the most comfortable position.

Around the joint are a complex set of strong ligaments, muscles, tendons, nerves and blood vessels. If nerves and blood vessels are involved in the dislocation, the casualty may complain of tingling, numbness and discomfort extending down the arm, sometimes into the fingers, and circulation at the wrist can be absent.

You may notice a visible displacement at the shoulder and for some the appearance of 'squaring off' with a hollow at the shoulder joint.

Elbow dislocation – Elbow dislocations can occur after a fall onto an outstretched hand, or from a direct blow. You will notice an obvious deformity (sometimes a strange twist at the elbow) and swelling; this dislocation is usually extremely painful.

In severe cases, as with a fracture of the elbow, there is the potential for damage to nerve and blood vessels.

WHAT TO DO

Check circulation and sensation at the wrist and hand.

Treat the injury.

Shoulder dislocation – Immobilise the shoulder in the position of most comfort for the casualty.

If the casualty is holding the arm slightly away from the chest, pad the gap between the arm and the chest using spare clothing. Once the padding is in place to stabilise the shoulder, it is usually possible to flex the elbow (if uninjured), and bring the lower arm across the chest. Immobilise the arm here using an arm sling.   ...

Elbow dislocation – Immobilise the arm in the position that you find it.

Pad between the arm and the chest if necessary.

Re-check circulation and sensation at the wrist and hand.

Treat as an **emergency** if: Pain is severe (pain score of between 7–10). Circulation at the wrist is reduced or absent. There is a change of sensation down the arm or hand. There are other associated injuries or you are some distance from your transport.

Dial 999/112 – request police – then ask for mountain rescue.

Insulate from the ground, provide shelter and monitor your casualty whilst you await rescue.

TOP TIPS

In the UK your task is simply to give reassurance, immobilise the limb, if possible offer pain relief and arrange evacuation.

If the casualty has recurrent dislocations of their shoulder they may be able to put it back in themselves or ask you to assist them.

Problems with nerves in shoulder dislocations are common.

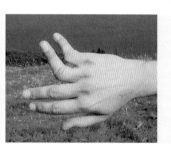

Photo: Keswick Mountain
Rescue Team

FINGER AND TOE DISLOCATIONS

Finger dislocations usually happen when the finger is forcibly bent, for example during a fall.

Toes usually dislocate as a result of a direct blow. This can happen if the casualty is wearing thin footwear and stubs the toe.

The joint will be misshapen, swollen, and painful. Once evacuated these injuries need to be assessed properly in hospital.

WHAT TO DO

Fingers – Place thin padding between the digits then tape to the adjacent finger. If grossly deformed simply protect and immobilise.

Place the hand in an elevated sling.

Toes – Pad between toes and secure to an adjacent one.

It may be possible for the casualty to walk on a dislocated toe, though it is painful and their progress will be slow. Be guided by the casualty.

Evacuate, then take to hospital.

TOP TIPS

I have witnessed several casualties instinctively putting a finger dislocation back in as soon as it happened, by pulling the finger back in line. This is not generally recommended as there could be other damage associated with this type of dislocation including fractures and torn ligaments.

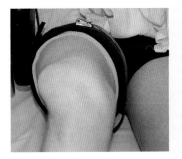

Photo: Mr Tony Smith
(North Wales Knee Clinic)

KNEECAP (PATELLA) DISLOCATION

Dislocated kneecaps usually happen following a sudden twist, or change of direction or a direct blow to the kneecap. Kneecaps dislocate outwards and end up to the side of the knee. Women are more at risk than men, often with a history of it happening before.

Once the kneecap is out, the casualty is unable to walk and is usually sitting on the ground with the knee bent slightly. In pain.

In the remote setting this is one of the few dislocations which is considered, by specialists in the medical field, safe for the non-medically trained persons to put back in. However the casualty is usually reluctant to let anyone touch it!

WHAT TO DO

If the casualty will allow you to touch the kneecap:

One person technique – Straighten the leg with one hand and gently push the kneecap back into place with the thumb of your other hand.   ...

Two person technique – One person holds the ankle, whilst the other places both thumbs under the kneecap.

As the person at the ankle slowly pulls the leg straight, the other gently pushes the kneecap back into place (if this fails or is too painful, stop).

If the casualty will not allow you to touch the kneecap or you don't feel confident about trying to put it back in:

Leave the leg in the position most comfortable for the casualty and call for help.

If the kneecap goes back in, it can remain unstable for some time. However if the distance is not too far it may be possible to strap the knee with a strong support bandage (or splint) and carefully walk your casualty from the remote setting. Be guided by what your casualty says they are able or unable to do. Then seek medical help.

If necessary call for assistance:

Dial 999/112 – request police – then ask for mountain rescue.

Insulate from the ground, provide shelter and monitor your casualty whilst you await rescue.

TOP TIP

If the kneecap goes back in this injury benefits from 10 minutes of ice treatment if available.

Recurring dislocations

REAL
LIFE
STORY

Once a joint becomes dislocated it is more likely to happen again. Some casualties are able to put their dislocations back in and may ask you to assist them in doing so. Be guided by your casualty. You should not routinely reduce dislocations; you can do more harm than good!

Dislocated kneecap

We were having a great day out; it was warm, sunny and everyone was in good spirits. On the way back towards the car I jumped down onto the path and landed awkwardly, I just crumpled into a heap on the floor. When everyone stopped laughing I found I was actually in a lot of pain and couldn't move.   ...

Looking down I was shocked to see my leg bent with a lump protruding out to the side by my knee joint and a big hollow where my kneecap should have been.

This was the first time I had done this and no-one wanted to touch it. Luckily we weren't far from the car. With painkillers and through gritted teeth, my mates managed to get me upright and carry me there, shoved me in the front seat and drove me to hospital.

Once the kneecap was back in place I was surprised by how much swelling there was (3 times the size). I had severely over-stretched the inside ligament so the kneecap was now very unstable. I had bandages put on for two weeks until the swelling went down enough to put on a full cast.

Since then I have dislocated my kneecap three more times. The last time was on a three-day camping and walking trip. Fortunately though, it went back in on its own as I was in the process of standing up to get a cup of coffee, and was straightening my own leg. We had no ice, so used a spare T-shirt drenched in a stream and bandaged that around the knee joint to provide some cold therapy and support. With plenty of painkillers and some physical help we made it back to camp. It was decision time; to evacuate or continue? Of course I chose the latter. I managed to keep hobbling around for another two days and although in pain, I made it though the weekend with the help of painkillers, friends and walking poles.

First thing Monday morning I took myself off to the local A&E, where I received a telling off for not going sooner.

Mandi Shipton

Sprains and strains

Soft tissue – ligaments, muscles and tendons – can become damaged as a result of a fracture or dislocation, or on occasions in isolation. The urban approach to managing this type of injury is the **RICE** treatment (**R**est, **I**ce the injury, **C**ompression with a bandage, **E**levation above the level of the heart). Finding ice to cool an injury in the remote setting may be difficult; however you may be able to use water from a mountain stream.

Sprain

When a joint is forced beyond its normal range of movement, the ligaments that support the joint can become torn or damaged; this is referred to as a sprain. It can be difficult to tell a severe sprain from a fracture; so don't bother trying. If the casualty is unable to move or weight bear on the injury, then treat it as a fracture. Sprains are commonly seen in ankles and the question many people ask is "do I take the boot off, or leave it on?" If you leave it on and they can walk, it might be prudent to self-evacuate the casualty then assess the injury when you are back at your vehicle. If you take the boot off, you may end up with an ankle so swollen they are unable to get it back on and you will now have to call for assistance. It's your choice!

LOOK OUT FOR

Pain.

Tenderness.

Swelling and bruising.

Stiffness and inability to use the limb.

WHAT TO DO

Minor sprains – Treat using the **RICE** method and/or apply a splint over the footwear and secure in place to offer additional support while they walk.

Severe sprains – If the pain is intense and the casualty is unable to use the limb, treat as a fracture; immobilise and splint.

If the casualty is unable to walk you may have to call for assistance:

Dial 999/112 – request police – then ask for mountain rescue.

Insulate from the ground, provide shelter and monitor your casualty while you await rescue.

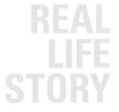

Torn ligament

I was racing in the Rhobell Fawr fell race which starts on a good track then goes into rough ground all the way up to the summit (734m). The descent is via the same route, and this was where it happened.

I had just circled the cairn on the top and was ready for a storming descent, but within 100m I landed awkwardly on a rock and the right ankle turned severely.   ...

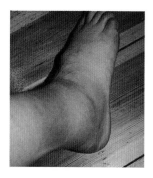

Photo: www.runsnowdonia.co.uk

Simon, racing alongside, heard it go – as did I. A sharp 'ping' accompanied by agonising pain. But I was racing, and the pain was quickly replaced with the fear of a DNF (did not finish!), coupled with adrenaline. However by the time I reached the good track with another 2 miles to go, the pain had set in. My ankle was so swollen by this stage that it was difficult to flex my foot. I gritted my teeth and figured it was either walk back or run back, so I ran.

At the finish I was in quite a bit of pain and was kindly helped by a few mates into the river where I 'iced' the injury. The minute I removed my shoe it was all over – walking that is. The shoe was most likely providing my stability. Due to the 'ping' noise I got an X-ray, which thankfully confirmed no broken bones; however my physiotherapist later diagnosed a torn ligament, which apparently can make such a noise!

Sarah Ridgway

Strains

When a muscle or tendon is overstretched, the fibres can tear or become damaged; this is referred to as a strain or 'pulled muscle'. These can vary from fairly mild, when the muscle is tender and painful, through to a complete tear when the muscle is no longer able to function. Simple muscle strains can be managed like sprains, using the **RICE** method of treatment. In severe cases where the casualty is in significant pain, and can no longer use the limb, treat as a fracture.

9. HEAD, SCALP, FACE AND EYE INJURIES

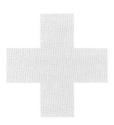

Any reduced level of response as a result of a blow to the head means the brain has been injured and, in the remote setting, is often treated over-cautiously because of the possibility of a neck or spinal injury. The term 'head injury' is commonly used to cover a whole spectrum of different types of injuries and can be confused with a wound to the scalp or face. For the purpose of the first part of this chapter the term 'head injury' refers specifically to a brain injury and not to other forms of soft tissue or facial injuries, which will be dealt with separately.

NECK OR SPINAL INJURY?

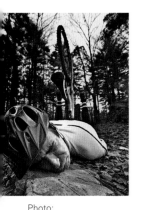

Photo:
www.istockphoto.com

Any injury to the head, or face, has the potential to create a neck (spinal) injury. In some instances it may be obvious that the injury is so superficial that a possible spinal injury may be extremely unlikely; in others it may not be that clear cut. Always look at the mechanisms of injury – what exactly happened – to help you work out the possibility of a neck or spinal injury.

Head injury – traumatic brain injury (TBI)

Head injuries occur through some form of **direct** impact – either something hits, or the casualty bangs, their head – or **indirectly** when the brain is bashed around inside the skull and becomes injured. In some instances, the casualty may suffer from both direct and indirect injuries.

Head injuries are categorised as mild, moderate or severe, depending on the amount of damage to the brain.

Mild head injury – concussion

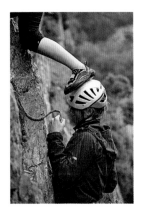

The concern for the first aider is that what appears initially to be a minor head injury could over time develop into something much more serious and life-threatening.

The brain is the consistency of egg custard and sits snugly – surrounded by fluid – within the enclosed bony skull. Concussion is a result of a blow to the head which causes the brain to bash against the inside of the skull. A casualty with a minor head injury is usually **A**lert (**A** of **AVPU**) and experiences a momentary disruption of their mental function.

It is a cause for concern if the brain does not start functioning properly fairly quickly after the accident. Continual disorientation and not being able to retain new memories – for instance the casualty forgets what is happening from one minute to the next – is **not** a good sign. Significant memory loss (amnesia) of events before the accident is also a concern. The mountain biker who struck his head and now doesn't know where he is, how he got there, or even who he is, has a more significant brain injury than the casualty who can't remember the accident but remembers everything before and since.

LOOK OUT FOR

After a blow to the head the casualty may experience some of the following symptoms:

Speaks of seeing 'stars' or some other form of visual disturbance.

Memory loss.

Headache.

Dizziness.

Nausea.

Confusion.

Complains of tiredness.

Moodiness, short temper or irritability.

WHAT TO DO

Establish exactly what happened.

Check level of response (AVPU).

Establish symptoms – a casualty complaining of pain in the neck should be treated as a possible spinal injury.   ...

Observe the casualty. Regularly monitor vital signs: level of response (AVPU), breathing and pulse.

For a casualty reporting any pain in the neck, or the following symptoms get **worse**:

Headache.

Vomiting.

Confusion.

Reduced level of response.

Double vision.

Dial 999/112 – request police – then ask for mountain rescue.

Insulate from the ground, provide shelter and monitor vital signs: level of response (AVPU), breathing and pulse waiting, while for rescue.

Head injuries and children: special considerations

There has been a notable increase in the number of children being taken into remote environments.

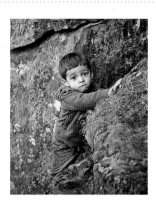

Research indicates that after a head injury the developing brains of children and adolescents may need longer periods of full rest in order to recover, compared to adults. It is common for children who have experienced even a minor head injury to have difficulties with memory and concentration. They can often feel tired and experience dizziness; you may notice changes in their general behaviour.

Moderate and severe head injuries

Anyone with a reduced level of response from a head injury should give you cause for concern. A casualty who only responds to **V**oice stimulus is said to have a moderate head injury, those only responding to **P**ain or **U**nresponsive are categorised as severe.

The first line of defence for the brain is the bony skull, and if the forces involved are significant enough, the skull can fracture. Within the context of the remote environment a fractured skull can be quite difficult to detect, unless it is a depressed fracture with an obvious dent. The typical signs of a fractured bone, such as pain and tenderness, are sometimes masked by other injuries to the scalp.

There is no specific treatment for a skull fracture outside the hospital environment. These casualties should be treated as for any head injury, with the added consideration (in view of the considerable forces involved) of possible damage to the neck and spine.

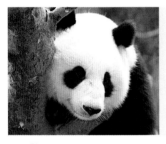

Photo:
www.istockphoto.com

SKULL FRACTURE

Fractures at the base of the skull may result in bruising behind the ear (late sign), black eyes – also known as racoon or panda eyes – and the fluid which surrounds the brain leaking out of the nose or ears. This fluid is recognisable by its watery, straw coloured appearance which, unlike blood, does not clot – and apparently tastes salty!

After any injury to the head the brain can bruise and swell. There could be bleeding into or around the brain (which can cause a build up of pressure) thereby compressing the brain (cerebral compression); this is rare but serious. Because the brain has nowhere to expand, the pressure inside the skull increases to such a degree that the brain becomes squashed, and is no longer able to function properly. The casualty will die if this pressure is not reduced, and quickly. A casualty with this type of head injury may recover normally at first (concussion) then, after a period of time, shows a reduced level of response and eventually becomes unconscious.

LOOK OUT FOR

Headache gets worse and doesn't go away.

Reduced level of response.

Suspicion of skull fracture.

Continued vomiting.

Continued memory loss.

Any seizures or fits.

Strange behaviour – confused, aggressive, irrational, appears drunk, excessively sleepy.

Loss of strength, movement or feeling down one side of the face or body.

...

Problems understanding, speaking or has slurred speech.

Strong slow pulse, and slow loud deep breathing.

Unequal pupils.

Also consider:

Is your casualty over 65 or under 5?

Do they have a history of bleeding or clotting disorders?

Are they currently on medication that thins the blood (e.g. warfarin)?

WHAT TO DO

If you think your casualty has a moderate or severe head injury:

Dial 999/112 – request police – then ask for mountain rescue.

Support and reassure the casualty in a comfortable resting position, usually with the head slightly elevated. If unconscious, place in a safe airway position.

Maintain the neck in a neutral position, as a spinal injury cannot be excluded.

Insulate from the ground, provide shelter and monitor the vital signs: level of response (AVPU), breathing and pulse.

With a significant head injury it is suggested you monitor the casualty's vital signs every five minutes. Record this and all relevant information about the casualty on your **casualty report form**, and hand it to the rescue services when they arrive.

Scalp injuries

The most striking thing about a scalp injury is often the alarming amount of blood. Treatment is no different from that of any skin or soft tissue wounds; apply gentle continuous pressure on the edges of the wound. This can be done using gloved fingers, or with gauze from a first aid kit. If pressure is applied continually for a few minutes, the vast majority of bleeds should stop. Only when the bleeding has been controlled should you dress the wound. Avoid over examination of scalp injuries; interference with matted hair and blood clots can often restart bleeding.

CLOSING A SCALP WOUND

Place a wound closure strip (or similar type of tape) over the wound, with the sticky side up. Take two strands of hair, either side of the cut, twirl them in the fingers and tie them in a knot.

Once the hair is tied in a knot bring the sides of the wound closure strips upwards and stick them together.

Tying hair can temporarily close a scalp wound.

Photos: Brian Wills

Repeat along the wound. Secure a dressing on top.

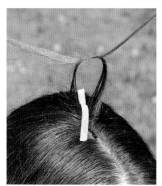
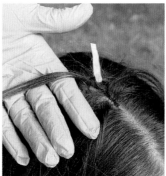
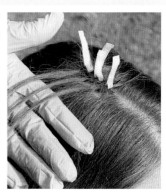

Facial injuries: wounds to the face

The face has a better blood supply than most other areas of the body, and heals faster. The general care of facial wounds is no different from the same types of wounds found elsewhere on the body. They can, however, look quite dramatic and as a first aider it is difficult sometimes not to react. Remember the casualty cannot see what they look like and will read your reaction as an indicator of how bad the injury is.

Even minor wounds to the face can sometimes look quite nasty!

Photo: Matt Shipp

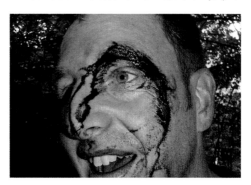

Facial fractures

Fractures of the face are uncomfortable but rarely an urgent problem – unless the fractured area causes an airway difficulty – and there is very little first aid you can do in the remote setting apart from maintaining an open airway and ensuring your casualty can breathe. With an unconscious casualty, a fractured jaw may cause the tongue to drop back into the throat, completely blocking the airway and stopping the casualty from breathing. Always place the unconscious casualty in a safe airway position.

Fractured lower jaw

The most common symptom of a fractured jaw is pain and if possible this should be controlled with painkillers. The casualty will experience difficulty speaking and be unable to open their mouth wide. Most of these casualties walk into hospital with no splintage (even when bones are broken in several places). Some support can be given if necessary with padding underneath the jaw. Your treatment and priority should remain with maintaining a clear airway, as these casualties often have damage to the gums and teeth and may need to continually spit out blood. The conscious casualty will probably be more comfortable sitting up and leaning forward. Casualties with facial or jaw fractures should not be made to lie flat if it makes them uncomfortable; their airway can become at risk. Where there are concerns about a possible associated spinal injury, the head can be held in a neutral position from in front or behind the sitting casualty.

REAL LIFE STORY

Fractured jaws, nose, cheek and eye socket

The rock, which was about the size of a baseball, came hurtling towards my face like an over sized bullet. The impact felt like a sledge hammer. Immediately I slammed to the ground, and began to feel the left side of my face fill with blood.

At first, all I could see was a bright white light, and then everything came into focus. I can remember seeing my brother's face, the look of shock, as if he had just killed me, which scared me beyond belief. I started screaming "my teeth! my teeth!" as I realised I'd been spitting them out.

I knew my face had to look pretty bad when I could barely see anything out of my eye, except for the outer corner of my cheek swelling, and the feeling of bones grinding against each other.   ...

Photo: Danny Thomson

My brother and dad helped to apply pressure and support with a jumper, and we made our way to the car, which fortunately wasn't that far away. I could tell both of them were panicking. The pain was excruciating and I found it really hard to breath.

Looking back there wasn't an awful lot of first aid to be done, apart from the jumper to hold everything still and mop up the blood. The only other thing that would have been really handy was if we'd been carrying painkillers.

The x-rays and scans at the hospital showed that my cheekbone, nose, both my upper and lower jaw and the bones surrounding my left eye were completely shattered.

Danny Thomson

Eye injuries

Eye injuries have the potential to be devastating and they can be very deceptive, so take a thorough history of exactly what happened. Understanding the mechanisms of injury can help guide you towards identifying the type of injury and the most appropriate treatment.

Eye examination

Look into the casualty's eyes and compare one with the other. Check the pupil size and shape, and compare the coloured part (iris), looking for symmetry (both eyes the same shape). Ask the casualty to move their eyes up and down, and from side to side, by following your finger and checking that they move in the same direction. Find out how much they can see in comparison to the other eye. Do this by covering one eye and then asking the casualty to read some written material, for example labelling on clothes or food wrappers. If they struggle to see words, ask them if they can see your hand movements. If they are unable to see these hand gestures, try to establish whether they can see any light.

Foreign body in the eye

This is a common problem in the outdoors, when small insects or dirt can end up on the surface of the eye.

LOOK OUT FOR

Symptoms may include:

The casualty feels something going into the eye, e.g. an insect.

The eye goes into spasm, making it difficult to open.

Foreign material on the surface of the eye, or under the eyelids.

The eye is red and watering.

Casualty feels like there is grit in the eye, or it is painful.

Blinking or moving the eye makes it worse.

WHAT TO DO

Sit the casualty down in a semi-reclining position.

Examine the eye carefully – look under the eyelids as well.

Whether you can see an object or not, try flushing the eye with normal saline solution.

If washing the eye doesn't work, try using a piece of damp gauze, or a clean handkerchief, to remove any object on the white of the eye.

Never touch the coloured part of the eye.

Repeat the process as necessary.

Chemical eye injury

Insect repellent and sun cream in the eyes can be a problem; but these are primarily irritants, which do not usually cause permanent damage. The eye lid becomes swollen and the eye itself is painful, red and burns. The single most important thing you can do is to irrigate immediately: wash the eye out with lots of water. Although saline is the best solution to use, any clean water is an acceptable alternative. The casualty will probably find they are unable to open the eye spontaneously, due to pain; you may have to gently pry the lids open with your fingers.

Penetrating and blunt eye injuries

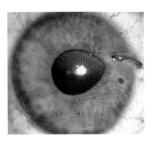

An obvious penetrating injury to the eye. Photo: Dr Chua Chung Hen

These types of eye injuries can cause significant visual loss. A blunt impact injury is the more common of the two and can damage the front of the eye, including the eye lid, lens, etc. and also the back (retina and nerves).

The eye is intrinsically a goo-filled ball, and when punctured the contents of the eye can spill out; however, in some cases these wounds can self-seal, making detection difficult. This type of injury can be caused by a high-speed foreign body, such as a stone thrown up while mountain biking at speed. A careful and detailed history, combined with a thorough examination, will be particularly important with these casualties.

A blow to the eye can result in a 'black eye' and/or bleeding into the white or coloured part. It is also possible to break bones around the eye or damage the retina (at the back of the eye). If you are at all concerned take the casualty to hospital to be assessed properly. Bleeding into the white of the eye is not normally a cause for concern, unless due to a severe injury to the eye itself, or seen in conjunction with a significant blow to the head. Bleeding into the coloured part of the eye, however, is usually serious.

LOOK OUT FOR

The symptoms may include the following.

Penetrating Injury	Blunt Trauma Injury
History of a high speed impact from something hitting the eye.	Loss or blurred vision.
Irregular shaped pupil.	Blood in the white or coloured part of the eye.
Obvious injury with 'goo' leaking out of the eye.	Unequal pupils – one much larger than the other.
Obvious embedded object sticking out of the eye.	Reduced movements of the eye.
The casualty reports being able to see shapes 'floating' in front of the eye when previously there was none.	

WHAT TO DO

Minor eye injury

Simply ask the casualty to keep the eye closed. Offer pain relief if you are able to. Evacuate from the remote setting then, if necessary, take to hospital.

Serious eye injury

Dial 999/112 – request police – then ask for mountain rescue.

If you think this is a serious injury (including penetrating injuries with the object still embedded), lie the casualty down, insulate from the ground, keep them still, provide shelter and monitor while you wait for rescue.

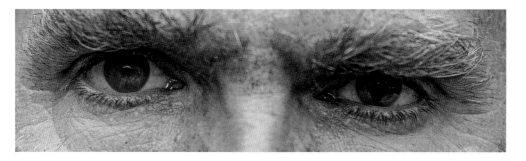

REAL LIFE STORY

Eye injury while gorge scrambling

A colleague and I were taking a group of teenagers down a gorge in North Wales. I set up a simple rope system, which could be released to allow them to swim out of a pool without being attached to the rope. I would let go of the system when they were just above the water, dropping them the last few feet. This proved a hit and all was going smoothly until about the sixth student when, as I released the system, there was a crack, the end of the rope shot up and I felt a blow to my eye.

I realised I had been hit, but there wasn't really any pain. I slowly opened my eye expecting to 'see stars'. I knew something was seriously wrong when all I could see was a red haze. What I remember was a sick, 'oh no' feeling. I called over to Chris, the other instructor. I could tell, by the look on his face, that it was serious and afterwards he said that he could see blood filling the coloured part of the eye from the bottom up, 'cartoon style'. We still had a group in the gorge to deal with, but they behaved fantastically when they …

realised what had happened, and we were able to climb out within the hour and make our way to Bangor hospital. I was still not in pain.

The eyelid had closed on impact and all damage was internal. I was in a hospital bed for a week, forbidden to walk even to the loo, in case of a re-bleed, and it was several months before they were prepared to operate. The injury, I was told, was similar to that caused by being hit by a squash ball in the eye, and resulted in the loss of my natural lens, and damage to the muscles which control the pupil. The lens was replaced by a plastic insert, and I now have a permanently odd shaped, fully dilated, pupil. It doesn't particularly affect day to day life, except that in bright sunlight I have to either close the eye or wear sunglasses. I am, however, very conscious that I now only have one good eye.

Rod White

Scratch to the eye

A scratch to the surface of the eye gives the sensation of there being something in it. The eye becomes very watery and produces blurred vision, which usually heals within 24 to 72 hours. The eye feels painful and is incredibly sensitive to light. This casualty benefits from taking painkillers and wearing sunglasses if available. It is important to monitor this injury for signs of infection and increased pain or visual changes; if these develop, seek medical attention urgently.

Glasses and contact lenses

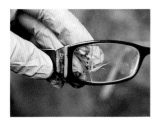

If the casualty was wearing glasses when they received their eye injury, these should be inspected and given to either the rescue services, or the hospital on your arrival. Contact lenses should also be removed but only by the casualty themselves if this can be done without applying too much pressure on the eye and only if you can be sure there is no rupture to the eye itself. If possible, contact lenses should be removed before significant swelling begins.

Eyelid injury

With any blow to the eye, it is possible the eyelid may become damaged. The lid performs the important job of spreading tears over the eye and keeping it moist. A dry eye can result in damage to the surface, leading to scarring and even blindness. Torn or lacerated eyelids should be cleaned with saline, returned to their original position and bandaged snugly into place. Because the injured eyelid must be kept completely still, it will be necessary to bandage the other eye closed to avoid movement, such as blinking. In severe cases this type of casualty will need a rapid evacuation to hospital. With a torn or lacerated eyelid, examine the eye itself carefully for any related injuries.

EYE INJURIES FOLLOWING A HEAD INJURY

Sometimes the eyes appear abnormal after a head injury (traumatic brain injury). Be on the alert for the following:

One pupil larger than the other.

Eyes pointing in the wrong direction, or not moving together.

Bleeding into the white of the eye (from a head injury).

The eyes do not follow your finger, when instructed to do so.

Bulging of one eye.

Record your observations, along with the time, on your **casualty report form.**

Ears

Fortunately injuries to the ears in the remote setting are quite uncommon. Generally speaking, they tend to consist of minor damage to the skin and should be treated accordingly. More severe wounds to the ear usually go hand-in-hand with serious head injuries.

Cartilage injuries

Injuries to the cartilage section of the ear (not the ear lobe) may need specialist closure in hospital as they are prone to developing into a 'cauliflower ear'.

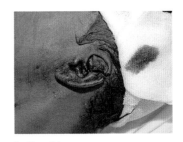

Cartilage injury.
Photo: www.istockphoto.com

Nosebleeds

Nosebleeds are common, particularly following minor injuries to the face or nose itself. They can, however, occur without any trauma – sometimes as a result of high blood pressure or anti-clotting medication – and in some cases be quite severe. Check if the casualty is taking any blood clotting medications such as warfarin.

Regardless of the cause, your main aim is to stop the bleeding.

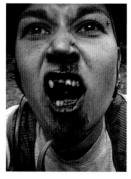

In the unconscious casualty nose bleeds and knocked out teeth (and subsequent bleeding) have the potential to block the airway if the casualty is not placed in a safe airway position.
Photo: Crissy Corner

WHAT TO DO

Sit the casualty down, tilt the head forward, allow blood to drain from the nose or mouth onto the ground.

Pinch the soft part of the nose for at least 10 minutes.

Ask them to breathe through their mouth.

The casualty must avoid blowing, or picking the nose once the bleeding has stopped.

If bleeding does not stop after 30min, or is exceptionally heavy:

Dial 999/112 – request police – then ask for mountain rescue.

Insulate from the ground, provide shelter and monitor vital signs: level of response (AVPU), breathing and pulse, while you await rescue.

Knocked out teeth

If an impact to the face knocked a tooth out, there may be bleeding into the mouth. As with any bleed, apply direct pressure over the socket using a clean handkerchief or gauze, and ask the casualty to bite down.

The complete tooth can be replaced in the empty socket; this should be done as soon as possible. Avoid handling the root of the tooth, if dirty rinse with milk (if you are carrying any!) or saline solution. Don't clean with disinfectant or let the root dry out. Make sure the tooth is the right way round then, holding it by its crown, push it firmly into the empty socket then bite on a clean handkerchief for about 15–20 minutes or until medical help is sought. Baby teeth or teeth that are in pieces should not be replaced. If the tooth will not go back in easily keep it in milk or saline, or as a last resort drinking water, then evacuate to medical assistance.

10. SPINE AND BACK INJURIES

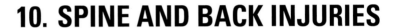

Nothing seems to strike more fear into the heart of a first aider than the thought of having to deal with someone with a spine or back injury. Most people are concerned about making a potentially serious injury even worse. Injuries to the back do not have to mean damage to the delicate spinal cord, nor do they necessarily leave your casualty paralysed. They can just as easily involve the nerves (which branch out from the cord) muscles, tendons, ligaments, bones (vertebrae), or damage to the discs which sit between the vertebrae. Spinal cord injuries leading to paralysis are actually quite rare in the UK. However, it is wise to adopt a cautious approach to any injury involving the back.

The spine

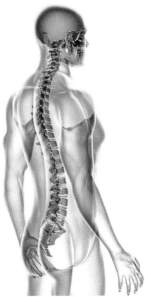

The spine can be divided into five different areas:
Neck (Cervical)
Chest (Thoracic)
Lower back (Lumbar)
Pelvis (Sacral)
Tailbone (Coccyx)
Photo:
www.istockphoto.com

The spine starts at the base of the skull and extends down to the bottom of the pelvis. It is made up of alternating vertebrae (small bony rings), which are divided by small flexible pads called discs – the body's version of shock absorbers. Down the centre of the ring-like vertebrae runs the delicate spinal cord. The cord is actually an extension of the brain and (like the brain) is protected by bone and floats in the same (cerebral) fluid.

The spinal cord is intrinsically an 'information highway', which makes communication between the brain and the rest of the body possible. The cord itself is made up of millions of little nerves, which branch out from each of the vertebrae to different parts of the body. Signals to start and control body movement come from the brain and travel down the spinal cord to the muscles. Sensory signals from the body are sent back up the cord to the brain. When the cord is damaged, the brain and body are no longer able to communicate, leading to a loss of sensation and/or movement (paralysis). The extent of paralysis will depend on where in the spine the injury has happened (known as the 'level of injury') therefore damage to the spinal cord at neck-level can result in paralysis of both the arms and legs, while injuries lower down the spine may cause loss of control in only the legs.

Vertebrae and discs work together to allow the body to bend forwards, arch backwards, and twist from side to side. During more strenuous activity the spine relies on strong ligaments and muscles around the vertebrae to stabilise and control movement. Photo: Malcolm Mills Davies

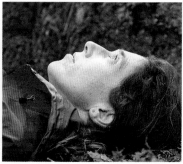

Managing a spinal injury casualty

Try to establish the mechanisms of injury (what exactly happened) and keep the casualty still – do not allow them to move. After your initial approach and assessment of danger you should take hold of, and support, the head and neck. With all suspected spinal injuries – conscious or unconscious – the head needs to be returned to a 'neutral position' (the head, neck and spine are all aligned) and held completely still; this is known as manual immobilisation. If the position of the casualty makes this impossible, support the head as best you can, and tell them not to move.

Neutral position, left: front view, right: side view.

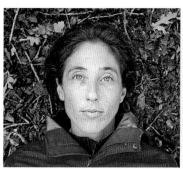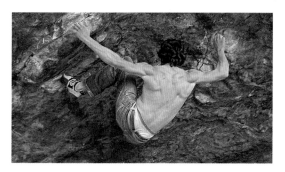

If while returning the head back to its normal neutral alignment the conscious casualty experiences any pain or increased tingling, numbness or weakness, or if you feel any resistance, abandon the repositioning and hold the head still in that position.

If you don't feel confident about placing a conscious casualty's head into a neutral position, don't worry, simply hold and support the head in the position you find it, and tell the casualty not to move.

Mountain rescue teams immobilise the head and neck using specialist equipment specifically designed for this purpose: a rigid collar **plus** full spinal immobilisation. Improvised collars are not recommended due to the unnecessary movement of the head and neck during their application; collars alone do **not** immobilise the spine. For this reason, the advice is to manually immobilise and support the head in the neutral position, until rescuers arrive with the appropriate kit.

Manual immobilisation of the head

Below are illustrations of different methods of steadying and supporting the head in the neutral position.

Casualty lying down

Three different methods of steadying and supporting the head.

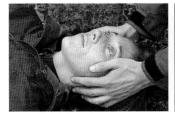
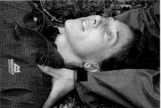
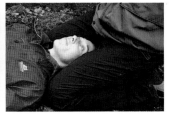

Hands either side of head. Try to keep the palms clear of the ears.

Hands on shoulders, forearms used to support the head.

Knees either side of head.

Casualty in a sitting position

Place the hands either side of head from the front, or behind, and hold it completely still.

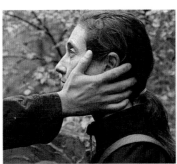
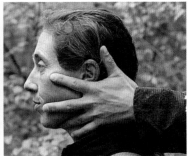

Because of the forces involved the suspected spinal injury casualty often has other injuries associated with the accident. It is important that you are thorough and systematic in your approach; follow your **ABC**s and undertake a complete head-to-toe examination. With cord injuries high in the spine (neck), it is particularly easy to miss damage to the abdomen and pelvis, especially if there is any paralysis or changes in sensation. Assess your casualty thoroughly, and constantly re-assess while you await rescue.

Photo:
www.istockphoto.com

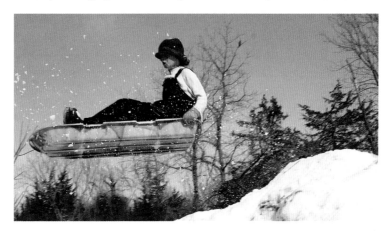

Certain types of accidents have a higher probability of a spinal injury than others. These can include falling from a height (particularly free falling), tumbling falls, high speed recreational and sports accidents (for example mountain biking, horse riding), a heavy object landing on the back or head, or a fall onto the back or head.

Spinal injury

Common areas for spinal injuries are the neck and lower back, and a number of these casualties often have more than one level of injury. After a fall any pain in the neck or along the spine should give you cause for concern.

Spinal bone injury (vertebrae)

LOOK OUT FOR

Pain at the site of the injury.

A step, or irregularity, in the normal curve of the spine.

Pain or tenderness in the skin over the spine.

Spinal cord injury

LOOK OUT FOR

Pain in the neck or back.

Loss of control of the limbs (movement may be weak or absent below the level of injury).

Loss of sensation or abnormal sensation (casualty talks of paralysis or a burning or tingling feeling, shooting pain, limbs feel heavy, stiff or clumsy below the level of injury).

Bowels may have opened, and the casualty may have urinated.

Pulse may be slow.

If the injury is high in the neck, they may have difficulty breathing or have stopped breathing.

Conscious spinal casualty

Having assessed there are no dangers around you or your casualty, try to approach the casualty from their feet end to prevent them turning their head to look at you. Ask them to keep as still as possible. As you assess their level of response (AVPU) by talking to them, take hold of their head and stop it from moving around (immobilise in the neutral position).

In a spinal cord injury other bodily functions may also be affected. These include an inability to control body temperature – the shivering response may be lost and blood vessels dilated – and in men you may notice penile erection.
Photo: www.istockphoto.com

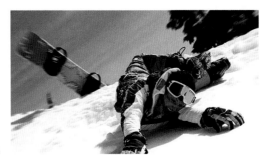

Primary survey – ABCs

If your casualty is able to talk the airway is open. If they are having trouble breathing this could be due to a chest injury, or a significant spinal injury in the neck; examine the chest to try to establish the cause. Check for any life-threatening bleeding before you start to look for any possible signs and symptoms of a spinal injury.

Secondary survey

With a conscious casualty, take a thorough history of what happened. Ask them if they have any pain in their head, neck or back. Find out if they have a history of neck or back problems such as arthritis or a previous break.

If there is a spinal cord injury the casualty may say things like, "I can't feel my legs," "I can't move," "Don't move me!" or perhaps mention a strange sensation in their arms and legs. Establish if there is any pain in the spine, change in sensation, weakness or loss of movement beyond the level of injury. If there is a loss of sensation, or paralysis, other injuries may be masked; so be thorough. Try to establish how much feeling and/or movement they have in their hands and feet, and compare the left side to the right; this is a helpful starting point (baseline observation) from which to compare future findings and is useful to the rescue services.

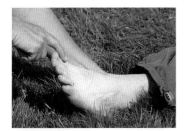

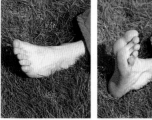

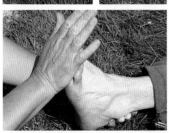

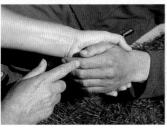

QUESTIONS: SUSPECT SPINAL INJURY CASUALTY

Did you hit your head, neck or back?

Does your head, neck or back hurt?

Can you feel me touching your toes?

Can you move your feet and toes?

Can you push your foot against my hand? (If a good effort produces no movement, or very weak movement, suspect a possible spinal cord injury.)

Can you feel me touching your fingers?

Can you move your hands and fingers?

Can you squeeze my hand? (Weak or absent grip on one or both sides indicates a possible spinal cord injury in the neck.)

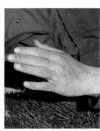

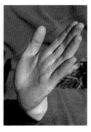

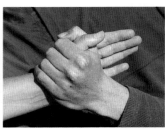

Photos: Brian Wills

If your casualty has full sensation and no pain or loss of movement don't be fooled into thinking they can't have a spinal injury; sometimes they can. Spinal injuries cannot be ruled out on the side of the mountain at a basic first aid level, therefore if the mechanisms of injury indicate there is a potential for a spinal injury, assume there is.

REAL LIFE STORY

Spinal injury

With hindsight I shouldn't have taken off that day. I wasn't in the right mind set, I just wasn't focused. I had to try out this new wing to get myself ready for the expedition John and I had planned for the Himalayas. It was quite a windy day; I was running out of time … the list goes on.

But I did take off. And fairly quickly I realised I should have spent more time setting up the controls, particularly the brakes, which weren't behaving like my usual competition wing. I came low over a boulder field, which with my other wing wouldn't have been a problem, but because the brakes were so different, I came in too low and just clipped the rocks. Because we fly with our feet supported in a sitting position, I impacted with my backside. I knew instantly I had seriously damaged my back, I was in excruciating pain. The only problem was, because I had clipped the boulders, I was still flying and despite my injury I had to land! I saw a boggy area and thought 'Oh well' and stalled the glider into the bog.

My troubles weren't over yet; the chute filled with air and started to drag me off towards more boulders. I collapsed the glider and pulled it towards me, trying to get everything under control, and me safe. I couldn't move anything apart from my arms. I didn't want to move either.

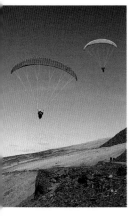

Photo: Brian Wills

The lads I was flying with that day, who hadn't taken off, came running over shouting the usual expletives. My good friend John arrived in a bit of a state, so I gave him something to do and asked him to go look for my sunglasses, which had flown off on the first impact.

I had fierce pain in my back and no feeling in my legs. I knew what I'd done and I told them 'I think I've bust my back'. As a first aid instructor myself, I had taught all these lads how to deal with this situation, so when I asked them to take my helmet off they initially refused! I'd trained them how to do this safely, and with a little persuasion they did a fantastic job, then immobilised my head.

Even though I was talking, the lads did an incredible job at checking me over, monitoring my breathing and pulse. Constantly re-assessing, checking if anything else was wrong. Really thorough!   …

I felt incredibly vulnerable. I desperately needed to know about, and control, what was going on. As a member of the local mountain rescue team myself, I had co-ordinated hundreds of incidents: I never thought I'd one day be trying to organise my own. Someone had dialled 999 and we were expecting a helicopter. The lads cut my harness off and cleared the area. They made sure the other paragliders were out of the air and packed away.

The news at the hospital was not good. I had four damaged vertebra. From my legs being totally paralysed initially, I did regain some feeling and movement in my left leg but nothing in my right. I'd also fractured my hip, but I didn't know that because the paralysis masked the pain. It's been a long road to recovery and, although now in a wheelchair, I still try to live as full and active a life as I can. And yes I did find my sun glasses.

John Gladston

Spinal shock

Spinal shock (better expressed as spinal concussion) is when the spinal cord temporarily stops working after an injury, causing loss of feeling and control below the damage. After a period of recovery, sensation and movement may return. This is the phenomenon behind stories of people being paralysed after a spinal injury, then amazingly being able to walk again.

Unconscious spinal casualty

If the accident has caused the casualty to become unconscious, it is fair to say that it may also have caused a spinal injury. If there was a witness take a thorough history of what happened.

Primary survey – ABCs

The priority of treatment remains with your **ABC**s. **A**irway on this occasion should be accompanied by manual immobilisation of the head and neck in the neutral position. If there are two first aiders, open the airway using a **jaw thrust**. However, if you are on your own, or you are unfamiliar with the jaw thrust, use whichever method you have been trained to use (usually a chin lift, head tilt). An open airway and effective breathing **must** take priority in the unconscious casualty with a suspected spinal injury: if they don't have an open airway they will die. **B**reathing and **C**irculation should then be checked and any problems identified and, if possible, treated.

Secondary survey

Complete a full and thorough **head-to-toe examination** (see chapter on **Dealing with a Conscious Casualty**) and identify any other injuries.

Pre-existing spinal injury

It is possible the casualty is already paralysed from an old spinal injury. You must be very thorough with your examination as this casualty will not complain of the usual signs or symptoms of pain and discomfort. Life-threatening fractures of the thigh bone and pelvis could go unnoticed.

Pre-existing spinal injury.
Photo: Challenge your
Boundaries adaptive MTB

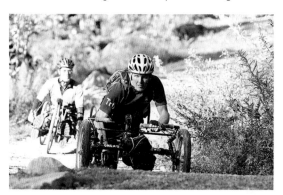

Safe airway position for suspected spinal injuries

Any unconscious casualty left on their back is in danger of two things; firstly the tongue falling back into the throat and blocking the airway, secondly the risk of stomach contents escaping up into the back of the throat, then the casualty inhaling the vomit into the lungs. For these reasons, no unconscious casualty should **ever** be left on their back. This premise is true for all casualties, regardless of whether you are staying with them or not! For an unconscious casualty with a suspected spinal injury, you should use the modified safe airway position. If the casualty has landed in a safe airway position (any position where the mouth is lower than the back of the throat) there is no need to move them as the tongue will fall forwards, and any fluid (such as blood or vomit) will simply drain away. Continue to ensure the airway is clear and open, that the casualty is breathing, and then monitor their vital signs until help arrives.

Modified safe airway position

The spinal log roll is a useful technique not only to place the casualty into a modified safe airway position, but also to treat other injuries. This should ideally be performed using five helpers and a lead first aider taking control of the head. The aim of the roll is to keep the casualty's head in the 'neutral position' then rotate them over keeping the nose, breast bone and genitals in one line, avoiding any bending or twisting of the spine. If the casualty has any suspected fractures of the arms or legs, these should ideally be splinted beforehand.

If you are on your own, use the normal method of placing your casualty into a safe airway position, while attempting to keep the spine as straight as possible.

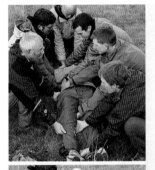

SPINAL LOG ROLL INTO A SAFE AIRWAY POSITION

As the lead first aider take control of the head and hold it in the neutral position. Place three people down the side you wish to roll towards and the other two on the opposite side. Lay the casualty's legs out straight.

Helper 1: (at the shoulders) place the casualty's nearest arm out of the way, and bring their other arm across their chest. Place your hand on the casualty's shoulder and your other hand on their waist.

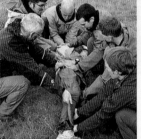

Helper 2: (at the waist) place your hand on the hip and your other under the opposite thigh.

Helper 3: (at the legs) place your hands under the opposite lower leg and ankle.

Helpers 4 & 5: (on the other side) place your hands under the casualty as shown.

On your command **slowly** turn the casualty keeping the head, torso and legs in one straight line. As the casualty is rotated helpers 3 and 4 can help to gently guide the casualty up, over, then down.

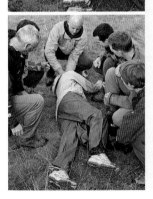

After turning the casualty over bend the uppermost knee and place some form of padding such as a rucksack underneath to stop any over rotation of the pelvis. Once in this position the lead first aid **must** continue to hold the head in a neutral position until medical help arrives. If you are on your own try to place some padding underneath the head before going for help.

Summary

WHAT TO DO

Assess danger then establish the casualty's level of response by talking to them. If conscious tell them to remain still.   ...

Take control of the head and hold it in a neutral position.

Primary survey

Airway: the conscious casualty will be talking, therefore the airway will be open and clear. For the unconscious casualty open the airway (if trained use a **jaw thrust**).

Breathing: is the casualty having difficulty breathing? Check the chest for injuries.

Circulation: check for and control any bleeding.

Secondary survey

Take a thorough history from the casualty (or witnesses) to establish the mechanisms of the injury.

Complete a head-to-toe examination; identify any other injuries. For the conscious casualty assess loss of sensation or movement in the arms and legs.

Place the unconscious casualty into a safe airway position: if possible use the modified spinal technique.

Dial 999/112 – request police – then ask for mountain rescue.

Insulate from the ground, provide shelter and monitor vital signs: level of response (AVPU), breathing and pulse, while you await rescue.

Record all your findings on your **casualty report form** and hand to the rescue services on their arrival.

Helmets

Many outdoor activities involve wearing a helmet, and there is a strong link between head injuries and damage to the neck and spine. Although helmets can reduce some injuries, they may not prevent them. If the casualty has sustained a head injury while wearing a helmet, check the helmet for signs of damage; this will give you some idea of the forces involved and any points of impact. If the helmet has been removed, make sure it is available to the rescue services who attend; the helmet should be taken to the hospital with the casualty. Any **unconscious** casualty with a head injury in the remote setting should be treated as if they also have a spinal injury.

Removing a helmet

Removing helmets can be particularly challenging, especially full face helmets. Careful consideration and stabilisation of the neck are important, and is best done with two people. It would be advantageous for anyone who may have to deal with casualties wearing full faced helmets to have practised this technique before they need to remove one for real.

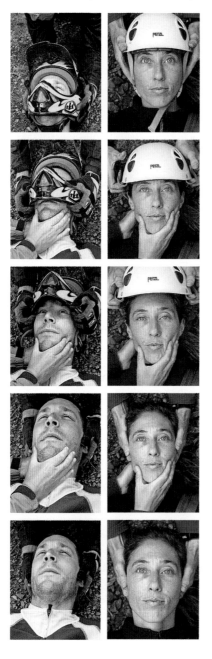

REMOVING A HELMET: TWO PERSON TECHNIQUE

The head should initially be held in a neutral position.

Undo the chin strap. The most experienced person supports the neck from in front - thumb and index finger of one hand on the jaw, and the other hand behind the back of the neck. The second person holds the side of helmet from above and pulls outwards, expanding the rim.

Continue to support the head from below as the second person removes the helmet in one smooth movement.

When the helmet is removed, the second person should take control and stabilise the head and neck in the neutral position.

Once the head is stabilised above, the person supporting the chin and neck can remove their hands.

Moving a spinal injury casualty

Never move a possible spinal injury casualty, **unless** they are in danger or you are unable to assess and open the unconscious casualty's airway, and then only move them the shortest distance possible. Moving a casualty with a possible spinal injury is dealt with in the chapter on **Moving and Carrying a Casualty.**

Back injuries

Muscular strain and spasm

A common back injury is a muscle strain. The pain and muscle spasm is located off to the side of the spine, as opposed to over it. The casualty needs to keep mobile, otherwise the muscle stiffens up and goes into spasm; avoid lying them down unless they are unable to walk. This casualty can be in considerable pain which, for an unlucky few, may be severe and completely incapacitating.

Ruptured disc (slipped disc)

Ruptured discs (also known as slipped discs) commonly occur in the neck and lower back and can be due to injury or degeneration from old age. Symptoms include severe pain in the spine, with muscle spasm which is worse on movement, and an inability to stand up straight. If the disc presses on nerves coming off the spinal cord the casualty may experience a shooting pain down the back of the buttock and leg (sciatica), or pins and needles in an area of one leg. A casualty with any abnormal sensation in the legs, buttocks or genitals should be seen by a doctor. Treatment includes painkillers, heat packs and keeping mobile. In most cases the pain disappears in a few days or weeks.

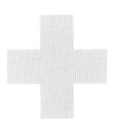

11. MEDICAL CONDITIONS

Acute medical conditions such as a heart attack, stroke or complications in pregnancy need urgent evacuation to hospital and every second will count. Problems arising from medical conditions such as angina, diabetes and epilepsy may on occasions be dealt with in the remote setting; however sometimes these will also require an emergency response.

Heart attack and angina

Heart attack and angina are both conditions of the heart. Heart attacks are acute and need to be seen in hospital urgently. Angina is a condition that can, on a day to day basis, be managed with medication.

Angina

Angina is a common condition caused by narrowing of the arteries that feed blood to the heart muscle. At rest the heart is fine; however when exercising the heart muscle demands more blood at a quicker rate, which the narrowed arteries simply cannot supply. This results in *temporary* chest pain, or discomfort. With rest alone these symptoms usually disappear within about 10 minutes. Combine rest with prescription medication (GTN – glyceryl trinitrate) and the symptoms should disappear in about two minutes. If the pain does not ease, or the symptoms are different or more intense than usual, the casualty may be having a heart attack.

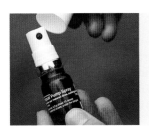

GTN – GLYCERYL TRINITRATE

GTN can be taken as a spray or tablet. The tablet is placed under the tongue and the spray is sprayed into the mouth. Once absorbed into the body it works by relaxing the blood vessels, widening the coronary arteries and increasing the flow of blood to the heart muscle.

LOOK OUT FOR

Pain, ache, discomfort or tightness in the middle of the chest on exercise.

Pain in the jaw, neck, one or both arms (usually the left) or stomach.

May also include:

Breathlessness.

Dizziness.

Nausea.

Belching (burping).

Restlessness.

WHAT TO DO

Ask the casualty to stop what they are doing and sit down.

Make them comfortable and give reassurance.

If the casualty has angina medication, find it and let them administer it themselves.

If the pain goes away after rest and/or medication the casualty may be able to resume their activity.

If the pain does not subside after rest or three doses of medication, or if the casualty looks ill, suspect a heart attack.

Dial 999/112 – request police – then ask for mountain rescue.

Insulate from the ground, provide shelter and monitor vital signs: level of response (AVPU), breathing and pulse, while you await rescue.

Heart attack

Heart attacks occur when a coronary artery (the artery that supplies blood to the heart muscle itself) becomes completely blocked, for example by a clot. Once the blood supply is cut off the heart muscle begins to die. The biggest danger here is that the heart may actually stop beating (cardiac arrest).

One symptom often mentioned in relation to a heart attack is chest pain: however in some instances the casualty may suffer no pain at all. These individuals are said to be experiencing a 'silent heart attack'; their main complaint may simply be a lack of energy, feeling sick and perhaps shortness of breath. This can happen with diabetics, as the casualty's condition may damage the nerves that transmit chest pain. However, any casualty who does present with chest pain should be treated with extreme caution, and a heart attack suspected until proven otherwise.

Mountain Rescue heart attack statistics

Age Range	Fatal	Non-Fatal	Total
10-19	0	1	1
20-29	2	4	6
30-39	3	10	13
40-49	27	15	44
50-59	66	48	144
60-69	78	56	134
70-79	37	37	74
80-89	3	10	13
Total	218	181	399

From Mountain Rescue England and Wales: 1996–2012.

Medication and heart attacks

Casualties suffering from a suspected heart attack may be offered soluble or dispersible aspirin (300mg); ask them to chew then swallow it. Don't be frightened to do this; aspirin can and does save lives, and the quicker they receive it the better their chance of survival. Soluble and dispersible aspirin is absorbed quicker into the body than a standard tablet. As with any medication, before offering aspirin ensure the casualty is able to take it and never give it to children under the age of 16.

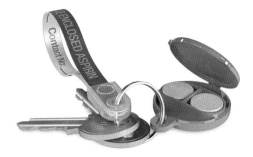

ASPOD. This handy little key ring keeps the aspirin (300mg) safely protected and always to hand. Photo: C-Beam Developments Ltd

LOOK OUT FOR

Symptoms vary from one person to another therefore the casualty may be experiencing some of the following:

Severe central chest pain; feels like a heavy pressure, tightness or squeezing.

Pain may travel into the jaw, neck, down one or both arms, into the back and abdomen.

Shortness of breath.

Feeling dizzy or faint.

Nausea and vomiting.

Skin is bluish in colour, pale, cold and clammy, lips may turn blue.

Profuse sweating.

Casualty is anxious and expresses a sense of 'impending doom'.

Looks very ill!

WHAT TO DO

Dial 999/112 – request police – then ask for mountain rescue.

Stay calm and help the casualty to sit down in a comfortable position – this is often a semi-reclined sitting position with the knees bent – and insulate from the ground.

If the casualty has angina medication, encourage them to take it.

If the casualty is able to take aspirin you may offer 300mg of soluble or dispersible aspirin which should be chewed and then swallowed.

Provide shelter and monitor their vital signs: level of response (AVPU), breathing and pulse, while you await rescue.

If they become unconscious, open the airway and check for breathing. If they stop breathing, be prepared to start basic life support (CPR).

Heart attacks are a medical emergency and require urgent evacuation. The sooner blood can be restored to the heart muscle, the better their chance of survival; this can only be done through advanced cardiac life support in hospital – not on the side of a mountain.

Heart attack risk factors

There are a number of risk factors that leave some people more susceptible to a heart attack than others. If your casualty has chest pain and one or more of the following symptoms it would be advisable to **dial 999/112** as there is a high probability they are having a heart attack.

- Male.

- Overweight.

- Diabetic.

- Smoker.

- High cholesterol.

- High blood pressure.

- Family history of heart disease.

- Previously had a heart attack or has angina.

- Engages in recreational use of amphetamines or cocaine.

Stroke

A stroke is the death of brain cells caused by a lack of blood flow, either from a clot or bleed within the brain. It is a medical emergency which requires urgent evacuation to hospital – the sooner the better.

The specific symptoms of a stroke will depend on which part of the brain has been affected; subsequently every casualty will present with slightly different symptoms. However to help you recognise someone who may be experiencing a stroke you can use the **FAST** method.

Think **STROKE** think **FAST**

Face Look at the casualty's face: you may notice a droop on one side of the mouth or eye. Ask them to smile or pull out their tongue; look for symmetry.

Arms Check for arm weakness or numbness: ask the casualty to raise both arms and keep them there. Are they unable to do this?

Speech Speech may be slurred, garbled or they may be unable to talk or find the right words despite being awake.

Time Time to call **999/112** if you notice any of these symptoms.

WHAT TO DO

Dial 999/112 – request police – then ask for mountain rescue.

Lie the casualty down, but raise the head and shoulders. Insulate them from the ground and provide shelter.

Observe the casualty's signs and symptoms and note if they improve or deteriorate.

Monitor their level of response (AVPU), breathing and pulse while you await rescue.

If the casualty becomes unconscious, place in a safe airway position.

A casualty who has experienced a stroke may find it difficult to speak; you must therefore find an alternative way of communicating other than through speech. A suggested method is to take the casualty's hands and ask them to squeeze your hand if they understand what you are saying. If paralysed down one side they may still be able to communicate through their non-affected side.

Some people are more likely to suffer a stroke than others (and the risk generally becomes greater with age); however a stroke can happen to anyone at any time, even children. If you notice a sudden change in the function of the brain – without a history of an accident or alcohol consumption – then you should be suspicious that this may be a stroke.

Mini stroke – transient ischaemic attack or TIA

If the casualty's symptoms disappear after just a few minutes, or hours, they may have experienced a transient ischaemic attack (TIA) or mini stroke. The brain has had a disruption of its blood supply, but only for a brief time. The symptoms are very similar to a full stroke; however they disappear completely within 24 hours. In a remote setting both the mini and full stroke will need immediate and urgent evacuation to hospital.

Diabetes

The food we eat is digested then broken down into easily absorbed elements – one of which is glucose (sugar) – which is transported around the body in blood. A chemical called insulin is released from the pancreas, which allows the body's cells to take the glucose out of the blood in order to create energy. In diabetes, the body either fails to produce enough insulin, or the insulin it produces does not work properly. People with diabetes therefore have an inability to regulate their own blood sugar levels.

Type 1 diabetic

Type 1 diabetics need regular injections of insulin throughout their lives. This can be done using a needle and syringe, or injection pen (insulin pen). In some cases insulin is taken using a 'pump', which is a small device usually strapped to the body that administers insulin through a fine tube leading from the pump to a needle sitting just under the skin.

The type 1 diabetic measures their blood glucose using a machine called a blood glucose monitor.

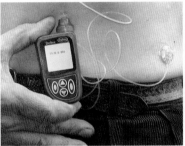 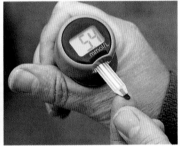

The advantage of an insulin pump (as opposed to an injection) is that it can help the diabetic to control their condition thus reducing the number of hypos they experience. Photos: David Hayward

To find out how much sugar is in the blood, diabetics use a blood glucose monitor. They prick their finger and place the blood onto a test strip which is then checked by a machine.

Type 2 diabetic

This is more common and is normally controlled through diet; being careful with sugar intake. However it is a progressive condition, which means the individual may eventually need to take insulin medication. Type 2 diabetics test their blood glucose levels by either monitoring their urine (checking against a coloured chart over several weeks) or with a blood glucose monitor.

Blood sugar conditions

Diabetics can experience one of two blood sugar conditions – either too much sugar in the blood (hyperglycaemia) or more commonly too little (hypoglycaemia). As a first aider it can sometimes be difficult to tell the difference between the two; if you are unsure treat them for hypoglycaemia, as you will do no further harm.

Hyperglycaemia – (high blood sugar)

If the blood sugar is too high, the known diabetic may well try to bring it down by the use of their medication and drinking plenty of fluids. For experienced diabetics who are trained, this is usually quite successful. If, however, the casualty is unable to gain control of their high blood sugar, or is too inexperienced to know what to do, they need to be assessed in hospital. Remember, a diabetic who has been managing their condition for many years will understand their diabetes better than anyone else.

LOOK OUT FOR

Drinking excessively.

Regular or more than average urination.

Excessive weakness/fatigue.

Blurred vision.

Strange smell on the breath similar to pear drops.

Drowsiness and if not treated leading into unconsciousness.

WHAT TO DO

If the casualty is unable to regain control of their blood sugar levels or you feel concerned about them:

Dial 999/112 – request police – then ask for mountain rescue.

Insulate from the ground, provide shelter and monitor the vital signs: level of response (AVPU), breathing and pulse, while you await rescue.

If they become unconscious, place into a safe airway position.

Hypoglycaemia – (low blood sugar)

Here the blood sugar has dropped too low and is often referred to as a 'hypo'. Diabetics can expect to develop hypoglycaemia from time to time, it is not uncommon.

LOOK OUT FOR

Mild

Hunger.

Muscle shakes and irritable.

Weak.

Pale sweaty appearance.

The casualty may appear drunk and stroppy.

Altered level of response.

Severe

Confusion and irrational behaviour, sometimes belligerent.

Slurred speech.

Seizures.

Unconsciousness.

WHAT TO DO

Where possible and if time allows, try to obtain a blood glucose reading before starting treatment.

Help the casualty to sit down.

If still conscious and able to swallow, give them something sugary to drink such as a carton of orange juice or sugary fizzy drink (not diet). If these are not available try glucose jells or chocolate.

If they improve quickly

Give them more complex carbohydrates to eat such as a biscuit or banana, allow them to rest until they feel better.

Help them to locate their blood glucose testing kit to check their blood (if not already located and used). ...

Monitor them until they have completely recovered.

If they do not improve

Look for other possible causes for their symptoms apart from diabetes.

Dial 999/112 – request police – then ask for mountain rescue.

Insulate from the ground, provide shelter and monitor and record the vital signs: levels of response (AVPU), breathing and pulse, while you await rescue.

Glucagon injection kit

Be aware that diabetics may carry an injection kit called glucagon, which is a pre-filled syringe for use in a hypoglycaemic emergency (low blood sugar). It is not uncommon for family members to be trained in its administration.

Glucagon is an injected medication used to quickly increase blood sugar levels in diabetics having a hypoglycaemic attack. Unconscious casualties usually return to consciousness within 5–20 minutes of receiving glucagon.

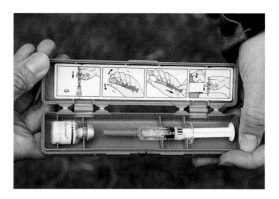

In a general context, a further point of note is that diabetics are prone to circulatory problems and as such they can be more susceptible to such conditions as frostnip and frostbite, as well as hyperthermia and hypothermia. Another concern mentioned previously is that diabetes can damage the nerves that transmit chest pain. It is possible therefore that a diabetic may be unaware of an approaching heart attack.

Seizures

Just like the heart muscle, brain tissue also has electrical properties, and seizures are basically a product of random chaotic electrical bursts of activity in the brain. There are many reasons why a casualty may experience a seizure (also referred to as a convulsion or fit). In serious cases, it can be a by-product of a significant head injury; on the other hand it could also be a relatively normal occurrence in someone who has the condition of epilepsy.

You do not have to have epilepsy to have a seizure. The following conditions can result in a seizure.

- Heat stroke.

- Head injury.

- Low blood sugar.

- Brain tumour.

- Lack of oxygen.

- Stroke.

- Infections.

- Certain drugs (such as alcohol).

- Lightning injury.

- Pregnancy (with complications).

- Poisoning.

If your casualty experiences a seizure and is not a known epileptic **dial 999/112** – request police – then ask for mountain rescue.

Epilepsy

If someone experiences a seizure due to epilepsy, it is rarely a medical emergency unless this is their first time, they hurt themselves during the event, the casualty is in a dangerous or exposed location, or if they do not come out of the seizure. The vast majority of epileptic episodes are fairly short (usually less than five minutes) and the casualty recovers quickly. Epileptics can control their seizures with medication and with a common sense approach can live normal active lives.

Most seizures occur without warning; however certain types of epilepsy (there are around forty different types) can give the individual a warning that a seizure is about to happen. This is referred to as an 'aura' and can happen far enough in advance for them to alert others, and get themselves into a safe place before the seizure starts. The outward signs can be as mild as a momentary loss of awareness, through to dramatic unconsciousness with uncontrollable thrashing movements. As a first aider you are most likely to become involved with assisting a casualty who is unconscious and experiencing a 'tonic-clonic' seizure.

LOOK OUT FOR

Tonic-clonic seizure – the following sequence is commonly seen.

Casualty loses consciousness suddenly and falls to the ground, sometimes with a loud cry.

They become rigid, contracting their muscles and arching their back.

Breathing becomes difficult, lips may become blue (cyanosis) face and neck may become red.

Convulsive rhythmical contractions begin, seen as jerky thrashing movements. These are in the back, neck and extremities. The eyes may roll upwards or off to one side.

Clenched jaw creates noisy breathing. Saliva may appear at the mouth, which may be bloodstained if they have bitten their tongue, cheek or lips.

Occasionally there is loss of bladder or bowel control.

Most seizures only last a few minutes, then the muscles relax and breathing becomes normal.

Casualty may fall into a deep sleep or come round feeling dazed or acting strangely (sometimes a little combative or aggressive) for a period of time, then slowly return to normal.

WHAT TO DO

Note the time the seizure started and make a mental note of what you see.

Make space around the casualty and ask bystanders to move away.

Remove any dangerous items such as hot drinks.

Protect the casualty's head from objects around them.

If necessary loosen tight clothing from around the casualty's neck.

Allow the casualty to have the seizure – do not restrain them.   **...**

After the seizure has stopped, open the airway and check they are still breathing.

If breathing, place them in a safe airway position.

Monitor the vital signs: level of response (AVPU), breathing and pulse, until the casualty recovers.

If appropriate record the duration of the seizure and a description of what you saw.

If necessary:

Dial 999/112 – request police – then ask for mountain rescue.

Insulate them from the ground, provide shelter and monitor their vital signs: level of response (AVPU), breathing and pulse, while you await rescue.

When should I dial 999/112?

- If they are not a known epileptic.

- Seizure continues for more than five minutes.

- One seizure follows another without the casualty regaining consciousness in between.

- The casualty is injured during the seizure.

- If the casualty remains unconscious for more than 10 minutes, once the seizure has stopped.

- If you believe the casualty needs medical attention.

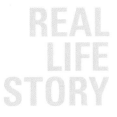

First time seizure, not known if epileptic

It was a beautiful sunny morning and we were all stood around procrastinating; chopping firewood rather than making a decision about where to go climbing. I felt a strange dizziness, much like when you stand up too quickly. My right foot twitched violently as I made my way from the log pile; something wasn't right?

The next thing I remember is opening my eyes to see my friend Chris, sympathetically telling me that I had just had a seizure. It was reassuring to see a familiar face, but I felt incredibly vulnerable and insecure. He told me there was an ambulance on the way.

Later, the paramedic asked how I felt, to which I said I was fine. He asked me my date of birth, and what day of the week it was, but I hadn't a clue. I took a deep breath on the oxygen, and tried to compose my thoughts.

Chris told me how my seizure lasted about three minutes, and that it was another three to five minutes before I came around. I had fallen onto my side, and all they could do was make sure I didn't bang my head. Beyond wondering how they were going to get the spittle out of their shirt sleeves, there really wasn't much more they could do.

Trystan Jones-Morris

SEIZURE DON'TS!

Don't restrain the casualty.

Don't put anything in the casualty's mouth.

Don't give the casualty anything to eat and drink **until** they are fully recovered.

Status epilepticus

This refers to a seizure that lasts thirty minutes or longer, or a series of seizures that happen one after the other without the casualty becoming conscious in between. This is a medical emergency, because during the prolonged convulsive stage the body struggles to take in and use oxygen.

Complications of pregnancy

Unfortunately a number of pregnancies terminate in miscarriages (roughly 1 in 4), with most occurring in the first three months. On occasions miscarriages in the early stage can result in severe bleeding which needs to be managed in a hospital environment. Any pregnant woman complaining of abdominal pain or vaginal bleeding should be treated as an emergency.

Ectopic pregnancy

Normally the fertilised egg travels from the ovary through the Fallopian tube and into the womb where it attaches and develops into a baby. If the egg attaches itself to the mother before it reaches the womb, it is referred to as an ectopic pregnancy.

In reality it is not easy to recognise this condition. Women at risk include any sexually active female of child-bearing age who has missed or is late with her period.

This is a life-threatening medical emergency because it can lead to severe internal bleeding. Women who have experienced an ectopic pregnancy say they had a sense that 'something felt very wrong'.

LOOK OUT FOR

The casualty may show some of these signs and symptoms.

Low or generalised abdominal pain which can be persistent and severe.

Nausea and diarrhoea (or pain when passing faeces (stools)).

May have vaginal bleeding which can be different from her normal period.

Light headedness, feeling dizzy or faint.

Signs of external blood loss or shock – including pale colour, dizziness on standing, a rapid weak pulse and confusion – and collapse.

WHAT TO DO

Dial 999/112 – request police – then ask for mountain rescue.

Keep the casualty lying down and resting; insulate her from the ground.

Treat for shock.

Try to be reassuring.

Provide shelter and monitor and record the vital signs: level of response (AVPU), breathing and pulse, while you await rescue.

Emergency delivery

Childbirth is a natural process that occurs safely in most cases. The mother's natural instincts will usually take over and lead the events. Apart from urgently requesting assistance, the only other thing you can do is to find a reasonably clean safe place in which she can deliver; then give her as much support and encouragement as possible.

During labour the mother goes through three stages. The first is when the womb contracts, the second when the mother pushes with the contractions to help baby out into the world and finally the third stage is when the afterbirth is expelled.

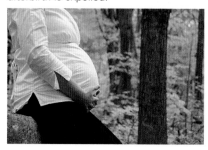

There is no reason why a fit and healthy pregnant woman should not continue to enjoy activities in the outdoors (with the obvious proviso of adopting a common sense approach). Photo: www.istockphoto.com

A detailed description of how to deliver a baby seems inappropriate here, as when push comes to shove it is unlikely you will remember what to do from reading this book! If you are going into a remote environment with a heavily pregnant woman it might be in your best interest – and hers – to familiarise yourself with the intricacies of having to deal with an emergency delivery. Alternatively you could call for assistance and then be guided by someone more knowledgeable and skilled on the end of a phone – this method relies on you having a mobile phone and being in a part of the country that has a signal. Good luck!

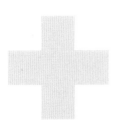

12. BITES AND STINGS

Anyone who goes into a remote setting will invariably come across some creature that has the potential to bite or sting. Fortunately in the UK there are only a limited number which cause us concern. First aiders should be aware of these creatures and develop an understanding and appreciation of their habitats, behaviour, and in some cases, their appearance and identifying marks.

Human and animal bites

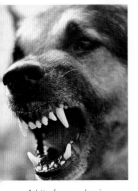

A bite from a dog is the most likely animal bite requiring first aid in the remote setting. Depending on the size of the animal, there is a distinct possibility of tissue being crushed, puncture wounds from teeth and, in more severe cases, tearing lacerations. Photo: www.istockphoto.com

Although there are unique variations in the characteristics of wounds created by different animals, the basic first aid treatment is much the same regardless of whom or what bit you. However, it is recommended that all human and animal bites are assessed in hospital, even if they look okay.

The vast majority of animal bites usually involve the extremities such as the hands, feet and face (including nose and ears) and carry a high risk of infection. Sometimes these injuries also contain foreign bodies (such as teeth) embedded in the wound.

WHAT TO DO

Stop any bleeding.

Thoroughly clean the wound.

Dress the wound accordingly.

Evacuate to hospital.

Never sew or close an animal bite with wound closure strips; these wounds are prone to infection and closure could cause complications.

Rabies

Rabies is a viral infection that kills. It has been around for many years and at one time was rife in the UK, after soldiers from the First World War returned to Britain with infected pet dogs. It was eradicated some time in the 1920s, and in the last 20 years only one person has died from contracting rabies within the UK; he was bitten by a bat and was himself an unvaccinated bat conservationist.

Snake bites

In the UK every year hundreds of people and an unspecified number of dogs are bitten by our only indigenous venomous snake, the adder (or viper). This section deals with the treatment of bites from this particular snake and not other exotic venomous snakes kept domestically.

The adder (Vipera berus) is not known for its aggressive behaviour; in fact they tend to be rather timid reptiles. Occasionally they announce their presence with a loud sustained hiss in an attempt to warn a potential attacker. If threatened, the front part of the body is drawn up in preparation for a strike. Photo: Emeritus Prof. David A Warrell

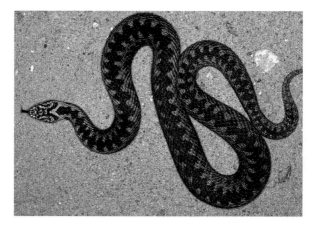

A bite from the wild UK adder – although on occasions very painful – is not generally regarded as particularly dangerous; children are more at risk of a serious reaction than adults.

Bites commonly occur between the months of February and October, although the apparent peak season is between June and August – just in time for the school holidays! Occasionally casualties are bitten on the toes or feet, although over half of reported casualties are actually bitten on the hands, many while attempting to pick up, or even worse, trying to kill the poor snake! Don't be fooled into thinking a dead snake is harmless; recently killed snakes have a reflex biting mechanism even after their death. So leave them alone.

Adder bite

One unlucky lad who was bitten by an adder was 14-year-old Jonathan Jones from Penygroes in Gwynedd. A warm sunny walk down a cycle track with his family during the Easter school holidays in 2007 very nearly turned into a fight for his life. Jonathan had stepped off the track into the scrub to retrieve a ball he had been kicking back and forth with his cousin. He's not exactly sure what happened next but thinks he maybe stood on the snake because, before he knew what was happening, it reared up, coiled around his leg and bit him on the ankle.

He described the pain as feeling like a wasp sting and noticed a small speck of blood, like the prick of a needle, where the fang of the snake had pierced the skin. There was only one wound and Jonathan assumed the other fang must have hit his training shoe.

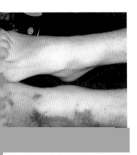

Jonathan's reaction
to the adder bite.
Photo: Carys Jones

After the encounter Jonathan continued to walk along the cycle track but noticed that his whole foot had begun to swell and turn red; he described the little puncture wound from the bite as turning into a little white circle. After walking for five minutes his whole leg started to swell up. His mum, Carys, became concerned and they headed for the local chemist for advice. Within about 10 to 15 mins Jonathan could no longer walk. He started to get red blotches all over his body, became dizzy, developed pains in his chest, had difficulty breathing and eventually started to lose consciousness.

He was rushed to hospital where his symptoms developed and worsened to include stomach ache and vomiting. Once it was established which type of snake had bitten him, it was a case of administering the appropriate anti-venom and monitoring his condition in hospital.

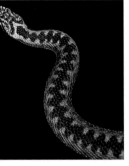

The adder is recognisable
by the bold zigzag
pattern down its back.
Colours vary from black
and white in the male
to shades of brown or
copper in the female
(some snakes are entirely
black). Males grow up to
60cm and females up to
75cm. Photo: Emeritus
Prof. David A Warrell

An understanding of this snake's behaviour and habitat can go some way towards preventing an encounter. Adders are found in a number of locations including rocky hillsides, sandy heaths, moors, meadows, rough commons, the edge of woods, sunny glades and clearings, bushy slopes, hedgerows, coastal dunes and stone quarries. They may also be found on the banks of lakes, streams and ponds. If you are going into any of these areas – particularly between June and August – be vigilant. Don't be fooled either into thinking that the higher from the ground you are, the safer you will be; even climbers need to be mindful.

LOOK OUT FOR

Around the bite area:

Pain and swelling of the affected limb.

Anaphylaxis – a severe allergic reaction (much less common), signs and symptoms of which are:

Throat and tongue swelling – the casualty may feel like the throat is closing up.

Increased breathing difficulties.

Feeling tired and weak.

Lowered level of response into unconsciousness.

Breathing and heart may stop.

WHAT TO DO

Identify the snake; if you have to go to hospital you will need to give a description.

Note the time of the bite.

Offer reassurance; a snake bite is a frightening experience.

Do not bandage! Avoid any interference with the bite wound.

If necessary pain relief can be offered in the form of paracetamol, **not ibuprofen.** If the snake injected venom it can cause bleeding/ blood clotting problems, and ibuprofen can make this worse.

Immobilise (splint) the bitten limb. If concerned evacuate and take to hospital.

Monitor for possible severe allergic reaction (anaphylaxis).

If symptoms of a severe allergic reaction are seen:

Dial 999/112 – request police – then ask for mountain rescue.

If swelling, mark the leading edge with an indelible pen and make a note of the time to track its progression.   ...

Keep the casualty still, lie them down and raise the legs. If unconscious place in a safe airway position.

Remove rings, watches and constricting clothing to avoid cutting off the blood supply as swelling progresses.

Insulate from the ground, provide shelter and monitor vital signs: level of response (AVPU), breathing and pulse, while you await rescue.

Despite what you see on television, **do not** cut and suck the venom out, tie a tourniquet around the limb, or apply a compressive dressing.

One final point is to remind you that adders are a protected species by law. It is illegal to kill, injure or sell these creatures. These beautiful timid reptiles need to be treated with respect; and remember statistically you are more likely to be killed by a falling vending machine than a bite from an adder.

Insect bites and stings

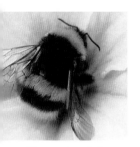

There are twenty-four species of bumblebee in the UK though only eight are commonly seen. Photo: www.istockphoto.com

Wildlife and particularly insects have the potential to enhance and intensify our experience of the great outdoors. They can also be a total nuisance, drive you to the brink of despair and for some people cause a life-threatening allergic reaction (anaphylaxis).

In the context of first aid, insects do one of two things, either bite or sting. Biting insects common to the UK include midges, gnats, mosquitoes, flies, fleas, mites, horsefly and ticks. Stinging insects include wasps, bees, hornets and ants. The sting felt is due to venom from the insect being injected into the skin; these insects are referred to as venomous and they attack as a defence mechanism.

A single sting from a native UK insect is more of a painful nuisance than a significant injury. However for those individuals who are sensitive to the sting there is the possibility that this can lead to a severe allergic reaction (anaphylaxis) and in some cases cause death. Multiple stings can also kill, regardless of whether or not the person is allergic to the sting.

Insect bites

It is possible not to even notice you have been bitten by an insect, especially if it was a tick. However some bites, such as from a horsefly, can be quite painful. Often the casualty complains of an irritation or itchy feeling over the site of the bite, which may develop into a small lump up to 24 hours afterwards. Usually this lasts for a few days before fading away. Complications may arise if the wound then becomes infected.

Ticks

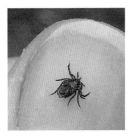

This little parasite is related to the spider family. Ticks can be as small as a pin head, or once filled with blood, as large as a baked bean and grey in colour. Photo: Katherine Wills

These disgusting little eight-legged critters spend their lives hanging around on vegetation waiting for the smell of a large mammal. Their intended hosts are usually wildlife and farm livestock and once on the host they embed their heads into the skin and feed off blood. Unfortunately humans and the domestic dog send out the same type of body heat and chemicals as livestock, which means although not their intended hosts, their next meal could be you, me or the dog!

As the popularity of outdoor activities such as walking and mountain biking has increased, so has the incidence of tick bites. Ticks like to hang around in grassy, bushy and wooded areas, and once on the host's skin, make their way to a suitable location, usually somewhere warm and moist. On humans they attach themselves in many places, but are most frequently found around the head, neck, armpits, back and groin areas. They are notoriously difficult to remove as they secrete a type of cement that anchors them to the skin. If not removed properly (and the head and mouth parts remain in the skin) the wound may become infected.

Tick removal

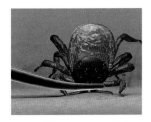

Tick tweezers avoid the need to get hold of the tick with your fingers in order to remove it. They have an excellent success rate for removing the mouth parts. Photo: The Tick Alert Campaign

The question of how best to remove a tick has turned out to be rather contentious, with a whole host of urban myths existing as to the proper and most effective method. Even medical professionals can not agree on a single approach; some belong to the school of 'slow pullers', others to the 'rotation technique'. Whichever technique you use, there are two key principles you should adhere to. First try to remove the tick without causing regurgitation of the tick's gut contents into the casualty; second, try to make sure its mouthparts come out at the same time as the rest of its body.

Manual removal of the tick will involve using your fingers to hold the body as close to the mouth parts as you can (protect your skin – if possible use gloves). There will inevitably be some pressure on its body which increases the chance of regurgitation into the wound. It is suggested therefore, when using your fingers, to rotate the tick which produces less pressure than a direct slow pull. An alternative to using fingers is to use a pair of specially designed tick tweezers.

Prevention

The only way to avoid being bitten is not to go into the areas where ticks live. They like to hang about in long grass, scrub-like areas and bracken, which provide the necessary humidity. They must have hosts to feed on, so there has to be an abundance of animals, and they need the right weather conditions; they cannot tolerate very dry or cold environments.

If you venture into their habitat then wear shoes or boots rather than open-toed footwear. Long sleeved tops, long trousers and long socks will also help, and light coloured clothing is better to spot them on than dark colours. Be 'tick aware' and check your clothes and skin after leaving their habitat.

TICK BITE DON'TS!

Don't use petroleum jelly.

Don't use nail polish remover.

Don't use a hot match.

Don't use petrol (especially with a hot match!)

Don't use glue.

Don't use alcohol.

Don't squeeze the tick's body.

Lyme disease

Ticks can carry dangerous diseases and one of the most harmful is known as Lyme disease, caused by bacteria that live in the saliva of an infected tick. Once the tick is on the skin and sucking blood, it begins to 'inflate' (become engorged). As it finishes its feed – usually after about 48 to 96 hours – the tick may regurgitate gut contents into the bite wound. Because the bacterium lives in the ticks gut it is important to remove it from the skin as quickly as possible.

Not all ticks are infected and accurate information on areas in the UK with infected ticks is difficult to obtain. 'Hot spots' in the country exist where there is a higher chance of being bitten by an infected tick. However, it is fair to say that tick infestation is on the increase and the best rule of thumb would be to assume any tick, anywhere, has the potential to transmit this disease.

Skin rash – 'bull's eye'

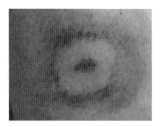

'Bulls eye'.
Photo: Katherine Wills

Many people believe that a skin rash is the first sign of Lyme infection. However it may appear at any time and for some not at all.

The rash does not have to have the 'bulls eye' appearance, as shown in the photograph on the left. It can vary from one person to the next, not only in shape but also size and colour. In fact, a rash of any kind can appear on any part of the body, even the scalp and for some, in multiple locations – not necessarily over the part of the body where the tick bite occurred.

LOOK OUT FOR

Some infected people have no symptoms at all, while others may show some of the following:

Rash – approximately 2–40 days after being infected.

Severe headache.

Muscle or joint pain.

Fatigue.

Nausea.

Facial palsy (paralysis).

Flu like symptoms.

Generally feeling very unwell!

WHAT TO DO

If any of the above symptoms develop within a month of a tick bite or a corresponding visit to a tick-infested area (you may not have noticed you were bitten) then see your doctor immediately.

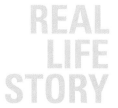

Tick bite

While in bed one night, I felt something on my stomach. I ran my fingers over the skin and discovered a strange little bump. I was in two minds about whether to get up and switch on the light or leave it to the next day. I chose the latter and, of course, promptly forgot all about it when I got up the following morning.   ...

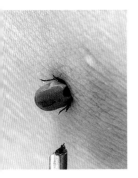

A tick embedded in human skin. Photo: www.istockphoto.com

It was only in the afternoon that something reminded me of the little bump. I pulled up my shirt to reveal a small black animal burrowed head first into my stomach with its hind legs sticking upwards. Fortunately, my companion came from Germany where ticks are common in the forests and recognised it, exclaiming, "It's a tick". I had read about ticks, but I wouldn't have realised that this was one. If I had been on my own I would have squeezed and pulled the dammed thing out there and then. But at least, once alerted, I knew not to do that. I used a plastic tick remover (like a tiny golf club). I slid it under the body of the tick around its neck and then twisted to safely remove the nasty little blighter, head and all!

Paul Gannon

Insect stings

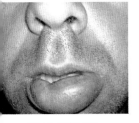

This casualty was stung on the lip while mountain biking. Any sting in or around the mouth or throat can develop into a significant problem due to swelling around the airway leading to difficulty breathing. Photo: Rob Booth

Insects that normally sting humans include the honey bee, wasps, bumble bee and hornet. The honey bee has a double-barbed stinger containing a venom sac which is left in the skin. This kills the honey bee but the sting will continue to inject venom while it remains in the body. Wasps and bumble bees on the other hand can sting multiple times, as they each have a smooth stinger that does not disengage from their body.

LOOK OUT FOR

Initial sharp burning pain.

Slight swelling around the sting.

Redness.

Soreness.

Warm to touch.

Anaphylaxis – a severe allergic reaction (much less common):

Throat and tongue swelling – the casualty may feel as if the throat is closing up.

Increased breathing difficulties.

Feeling tired and weak.

...

Lowered level of response into unconsciousness.

Breathing and heart may stop.

WHAT TO DO

Quickly scrape the stinger off the skin with either your finger nail or the blunt edge of a knife (only the honey bee leaves its stinger embedded).

Cool the sting site with a cold compress to relieve the pain.

If on a limb raise the affected part to help reduce swelling.

Consider offering pain relief.

Antihistamines (available over the counter) may also help.

Observe the casualty for 60 mins for signs of an allergic reaction.

If anaphylaxis is seen:

Dial 999/112 – request police – then ask for mountain rescue.

Treat for anaphylaxis.

Insulate from the ground, provide shelter and monitor vital signs: level of response (AVPU), breathing and pulse.

If they become unconscious place in a safe airway position and continue to monitor until help arrives.

Allergic reaction and anaphylactic shock

When considering allergic reactions and anaphylaxis it is important to understand the difference between bites and stings. Non-venomous insects such as fleas and ticks bite in order to feast on blood; as a consequence a casualty may experience a local reaction causing irritation. By contrast insects like wasps and bees attack (sting) as a form of defence, and their goal is to inject painful toxic venom. Allergic reactions are more common with stings than bites.

In the case of a sting, casualties usually experience a mild localised reaction around the area – swelling and perhaps blisters – which does not get worse and goes away over time. It can be helped by taking antihistamine tablets (available over the counter) but if the swelling is concerning, evacuate and seek medical help. More rare – but serious – is a generalised allergic reaction which can range from mild (including an itchy rash and some facial swelling) to severe in which the casualty experiences swelling of the airway, progressive breathing difficulties and becomes unconscious. A severe allergic reaction is called anaphylaxis and is a medical emergency. This is dealt with in the chapter on **Breathing Problems.**

13. HEAT AND COLD INJURIES AND CONDITIONS

The weather can present the first aider with two challenges: firstly it can be directly responsible for such injuries as frostnip and frostbite, as well as the conditions of hypothermia (too cold) and hyperthermia (too hot); and secondly the elements themselves can make treating and then looking after a casualty quite challenging. Understanding how the body responds to the heat and cold (and being able to recognise those reactions) is particularly important in remote first aid.

Body temperature control

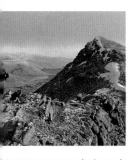

oto: www.runsnowdonia.co.uk

The human body tries to maintain a core temperature of approximately 37°C in order to function properly. The term 'core' refers to the major organs of the body, such as the heart, lungs, liver and brain, as opposed to the extremities such as hands and feet. The core temperature is maintained by balancing body heat produced with body heat lost. This delicate balance adjusts according to whether it is cold, wet and windy, or hot, sunny and humid.

HOW THE BODY PRODUCES HEAT

Exercise – About 75% of muscular energy is produced as heat.

Shivering – Receptors in the skin allow the brain to pick up the drop in temperature and trigger shivering as a response.

Eating – Food is broken down and digested, which in turn produces heat.

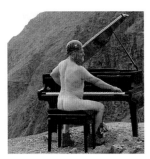

Photo: Mark Reeves

HOW THE BODY LOSES HEAT

Conduction – Heat is directly transferred to another surface, for instance the ground.

Evaporation – Sweat or water evaporating from the surface of the skin allows us to lose heat.

Convection – Heat is taken away from the body, through currents of air or water passing over it.

Radiation – Heat is lost into the colder environment around us.

We control heat-loss and heat-gain through either **voluntary** behaviour, or **involuntary** physical responses. Voluntary behaviour is consciously recognising a need and acting on it, for example putting on extra clothing when we feel cold. An involuntary response is when our body automatically reacts, such as sweating when we get too hot.

The body's involuntary physical responses are not very effective; voluntary behaviours play a more significant role in maintaining an effective core temperature. Unfortunately one of the first signs of an abnormal core temperature is often a change in the level of mental response, which produces poor judgement and a lack of common sense. If not recognised early and corrected, the problem is going to get progressively worse.

In an attempt to keep the core temperature 'normal', the body compensates by reducing blood flow to the extremities – such as fingers and toes – to limit heat loss. This deprives the extremities of warm blood, which then start to get cold, and if cooling continues, will eventually freeze, resulting in frostnip and frostbite. A casualty may experience both core and extremity cooling at the same time; if this is the case treating hypothermia must take priority, as this has the potential to kill.

Hypothermia (too cold)

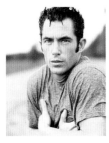

Photo:
www.istockphoto.com

Hypothermia is an abnormally low core temperature (below 35°C). In the outdoors this is usually a consequence of either prolonged exposure to the elements with inappropriate clothing, or exposure to the elements after the casualty becomes stationary due to an injury or illness (or both). The situation is often made worse by the fact the casualty is usually exhausted. In fact hypothermia and exhaustion frequently go hand in hand.

A wet and windy environment is worse than one which is cold and dry. Therefore in the UK the conditions for hypothermia exist throughout the year, not just in winter. A walker wearing only a T-shirt and jeans, caught in a summer thunder storm, is more likely to develop hypothermia than a well equipped winter mountaineer in a blizzard.

Mountain hypothermia – exposure

A common approach to defining hypothermia is to rely solely on the **shivering response**. However, in isolation shivering can be misleading because the body's reaction to cold is reduced in those who have a spinal injury, taken alcohol or tranquilisers, or those with a low blood sugar level. A more modern approach is to use the shivering response in conjunction with other signs and symptoms.

Hypothermia therefore can be loosely classified as **mild**, **moderate** or **severe**. Although categorised as three separate groups they are in fact a continuum moving from one to the next in which casualties may show certain signs and symptoms before others. The progression along this continuum can be potentially halted if the casualty is re-warmed.

It is important to note that in severe cases casualties enter a life-threatening stage, which may result in death.

Mild hypothermia

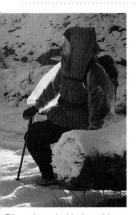

This casualty exhibits the involuntary physical response of shivering. At this stage, although depleted, the body usually has the capacity to fight the effects of the cold. Re-warm by providing shelter (emergency/group shelter), additional insulation, warm drinks and high energy foods. Once re-warmed this casualty can, with a little encouragement, be walked out of the remote setting.

Blizzard survival jacket: this sleeved, hooded jacket comes vacuumed packed into a tiny packet. An excellent addition to any outdoor first aid kit.
Photo:
www.blizzardsurvival.com

LOOK OUT FOR

Casualty says they feel cold.

Fast breathing.

Shivering.

Complains of tiredness, grumbling, mumbling.

Cold pale skin.

WHAT TO DO

Stop any further heat loss and gently re-warm.

Provide shelter (group/emergency shelter).

Insulate the casualty from the ground.

Put on extra clothes – change wet for dry.

Give a hot drink and hot/high energy foods.

Walk this casualty out of the remote setting.

Moderate hypothermia

This casualty has entered a very **vulnerable phase** in which rough handling can cause the heart to beat erratically. Their body no longer has the capacity to re-heat itself and shivering becomes violent and uncontrollable. The brain becomes affected resulting in poor judgement, confusion and irrational behaviour. No longer able to react appropriately to their environment they may start to remove clothes, resulting in a further drop in temperature. Handle this casualty with care.

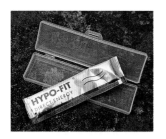

High energy gels are a useful addition to any remote first aid kit. They are excellent at providing the cold and/ or exhausted casualty with instant energy. They can also be used to assist a diabetic casualty having a hypoglycaemic attack who needs sugar urgently.

LOOK OUT FOR

Violent shivering which then stops.

Cold, pale skin, possibly blue lips.

Confusion.

Lack of co-ordination: difficulty using hands, fumbling, stumbling.

Becoming very drowsy.

Slurred speech.

Disregard for cold – jacket open, removing clothes.

WHAT TO DO

Treat as for mild hypothermia and monitor carefully.   ...

If re-warming has been successful and the casualty stops shivering then consider walking this casualty out of the remote setting.

If you are unable to re-warm you may have to **dial 999/112** – request police – then ask for mountain rescue.

Severe hypothermia

This casualty has entered a **critical phase** and is at significant risk of the heart stopping. This is a true EMERGENCY. Handle the casualty very gently and move as little as possible. Unnecessary or rough handling can force cold blood back to the heart sending it into a dangerous rhythm. The vital signs of breathing and pulse may be so shallow as to be undetectable. In essence the casualty appears dead.

LOOK OUT FOR

Shivering stops.

Unconscious (VPU of AVPU).

Cold, pale, blue/grey skin, possibly blue lips.

Muscle stiffness.

Shallow or no detectable breathing.

Weak, irregular or no detectable pulse.

Dilated pupils.

Looks dead!

WHAT TO DO

Handle very gently and move as little as possible.

Provide shelter (group/emergency shelter).

Insulate the casualty from the ground.

Place in a safe airway position.

Dial 999/112 – request police – then ask for mountain rescue.

Severe hypothermia and cardiopulmonary resuscitation (CPR)

The difficulty with a severely cold casualty who appears dead (with no detectable breathing) is that they may still have vital signs, you simply cannot find them. And therein lies the problem. The absence of normal breathing is usually the prompt to start cardiopulmonary resuscitation (CPR). However in the profoundly cold casualty if you were to start CPR you could turn a very slow, undetectable heart rhythm into a severely abnormal rhythm that can be life-threatening (ventricular fibrillation or VF).

The advice therefore is that in the remote setting with a severely hypothermic casualty for whom you cannot detect breathing you **DO NOT** start CPR.

Special circumstances

Because most heat is lost through the skin the relationship between the amount of skin to body size is important; this will influence how quickly heat is lost. Small bodies have a much bigger surface area to size than larger bodies; therefore babies, children and even small adults will lose heat considerably faster than larger people in the same situation.

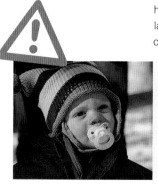

Walking with a child in a back pack to the summit of a mountain where the temperature can be below zero, will at times be little fun for the adult, and potentially catastrophic for a child. Photo: www.istockphoto.com

HYPOTHERMIA

Prevention is better than cure!

Wear and carry sufficient clothing for the weather conditions.

Wear clothing that allows ventilation, yet avoids excessive heat loss.

Stay dry and avoid excessive sweating.

Cover areas such as the head, neck and hands.

If the weather changes be prepared to change your route plan.

The better you know your group the more likely you are to pick up on unusual behaviour. Encourage every member of the party to be responsible for observing everyone else.

Eat and drink enough: watch for signs of poor eating in your group.

Remember that children lose heat faster than adults.

HYPOTHERMIA DON'TS!

Don't give alcohol to a hypothermic casualty.

Don't allow your casualty to smoke.

Don't leave a hypothermic casualty alone if at all possible.

Don't take off your own clothes and give them to the casualty if you are wearing them to keep yourself warm!

The most important tool for spotting hypothermia is an appreciation of the risks and an awareness of the signs. Remember, if one member of a group is hypothermic, it is possible that others are also on the brink.

Cold injuries – frostnip and frostbite

Frostnip is the name given to the early stage of a cold injury and if left untreated can continue to freeze, developing into frostbite (initially mild and then deep). With frostbite, the blood flow to the extremity is reduced and the fluid between the cells starts to freeze. Thawing then refreezing of this tissue can be disastrous.

Frostbite usually occurs in the hands, feet, nose and ears. There are two contributing factors. First the casualty is often hypothermic and has a reduced blood flow to their extremities; and second, they sometimes experience constriction in the hands and feet from boots being laced up too tight, over tightened crampon straps, or gloves that are too small.

The risk of cold injury is also increased in anyone who has consumed alcohol or illicit drugs, suffered previously from frostbite, has a circulatory condition such as Reynaud's disease, as well as those who smoke, have diabetes or taken sedative drugs.

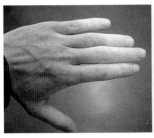

REYNAUD'S DISEASE

Reynaud's disease is a circulatory condition that affects the blood supply to the fingers, toes and sometimes other extremities. Exposure to cold is known to be a classic trigger causing the extremity to rapidly turn white, blue, then red. It is a common condition and is particularly prevalent in women.

Photo: Rob Johnson

On initial examination frostnip and frostbite look very similar. However while frostnip can be treated in a remote setting, frostbite can not. In reality many experts only categorise frostbite once it has been thawed and the damage becomes clear. It may be difficult in the outdoors to establish whether you are dealing with frostnip or frostbite.

Frostnip

Frostnip is the early stage of a cold injury (it is not actually frostbite) and is usually reversible within 30 minutes.

LOOK OUT FOR

Extremity looks pale.

Casualty complains of numbness and pins and needles.

WHAT TO DO

Flex the fingers, clap the hands, stamp the feet. Warm them up:

Place the extremity in the arm pits or groin.

Breathe warm air onto the injury.

The area often becomes red and painful, particularly on re-warming, with an accompanying burning feeling. At this point there should be no resulting long-term damage.

Frostbite – mild

If you fail to reverse frostnip, the extremity can go on to develop the early stage of frostbite, in which the outer layers of the skin and soft tissue are affected. The casualty will still be able to move the extremity as deeper skin layers, joints and tendons are not affected. The area often lacks sensitivity and subsequently is at risk to accidental damage.

LOOK OUT FOR

Affected part feels cold and possibly painful.   ...

Tingling, itching, burning sensation or numbness.

Skin feels hard, but the underlying tissue may feel soft and pliable.

WHAT TO DO

Stop as soon as the extremity goes cold and numb.

Find shelter, treat for hypothermia.

Treat as if for frostnip, re-warming using the body's own heat for up to 30 minutes. The casualty often experiences severe pain during the process of warming.

If after 30 minutes of re-warming the extremity has fully recovered, it is likely the casualty only had frostnip. However, if after re-warming for 30 minutes the extremity has not fully recovered, the prospects are much more serious and mild frostbite must be suspected. Protect the damaged area, evacuate the casualty and seek medical attention.

Frostbite – deep

This is a serious condition in which the skin, underlying tissues, muscles and sometimes bone are also frozen.

LOOK OUT FOR

Attempts at passively re-warming have been unsuccessful.

Complete loss of sensation – no feeling of pain.

If a large area is involved, such as the whole foot or hand, the tissue may appear blue or black, or red and mottled.

Caucasian skin appears waxy white, dark-skin appears pink or red.

If re-warming has occurred:

The area is extremely painful.

Re-warmed tissue does not look or feel normal.

There may be swelling, blisters and redness.

WHAT TO DO

While still in the remote setting:

Do not attempt any further re-warming.

Protect area from further freezing or physical damage.

If possible remove any jewellery from the injured area.

Dry the extremity and apply a non absorbent dressing – then wrap in a spare fleece.

Do not actively try to thaw the injury in the remote setting; get back to civilisation.

This casualty benefits from taking Ibuprofen 400mg if possible.

In the UK if deep frostbite is suspected in the feet:

Dial 999/112 – request police – then ask for mountain rescue.

Insulate from the ground, provide shelter, and monitor vital signs: level of response (AVPU), breathing and pulse, while you await rescue.

FROSTBITE

Prevention is better than cure!

Wear windproof, water-repellent clothing.

Avoid overly tight clothes, gloves, boots and crampons.   ...

Photos: Dave Hollinger

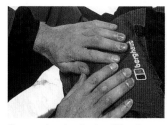 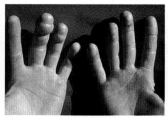 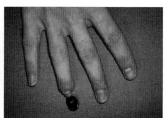

Fingers showing both mild and deep frostbite. Until the fingers have been re-warmed it is impossible to say how deeply frostbitten they are.

The development of blisters. These usually appear within a few hours after rapid re-warming. The blisters often do not extend to the very ends of the fingers or toes.

Amputation. Eventually the tip of the third finger on the right hand was lost. Tissue that has been destroyed usually hardens and turns black within a few weeks then self-amputates over 3 to 6 months.

Ensure everyone has sufficient food, drink and extra clothing, especially hats and gloves.

Wear gaiters to keep snow out of boots.

While on expedition, ensure you change socks frequently to keep feet dry – carry spare socks.

Stop and warm hands and feet as soon as they begin to feel cold or lose feeling.

If leading a group, set up a buddy system and watch each other's cheeks, nose and ears for signs of early frostbite.

Avoid smoking and alcohol.

Treating deep frostbite

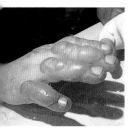

After re-warming **never** burst blisters and, if necessary, lightly dress and elevate the limb. The use of aloe vera is said to be particularly beneficial.
Photo: Rachel Griffin

Re-warming **deep** frostbite should **never** be done in a remote setting: thawed frostbite is a high risk wound that needs to be managed very carefully. The advice from the UK Frostbite Advisory Service is that this injury should be dealt with in a place where the skills, knowledge, strong pain-killers and other medication and equipment are available. In an ideal world this would be in a hospital experienced in handling deep frostbite injuries. However, in extreme winter conditions, such as those encountered in recent UK winters – with snow closing many roads – it may not be immediately possible to get to a hospital. The advice therefore would be to re-warm the extremities at the earliest opportunity then seek further medical attention when possible.

In this exceptional circumstance, a deeply frostbitten extremity should be re-warmed as rapidly as possible by immersing in warm water (40°C–42°C), – if you don't have a thermometer, use 'baby bath' water temperature (check with your elbow!) – for at least 30 minutes or until the limb is re-warmed, pliable and a red-purple colour (if available add a disinfectant to the water).

Make sure the injured area does not touch the sides of the container holding the water and continually monitor the water temperature. Re-warming the frostbitten injury will be **extremely** painful and pain relief is recommended: if available 400mg of Ibuprofen every 12 hours. Once thawed, protect the area using loose dry bandages and plenty of padding.

If you are concerned about the injury – whether you have been treated at a hospital or been forced to re-warm the frostbite yourself – you can contact the UK Frostbite Advisory Service. Digital photographs of the injuries can be emailed to the panel of specialists, who can advise you accordingly (go to www.thebmc.co.uk/medical).

FROSTBITE DON'TS!

Don't rub, beat or cover the frostbitten area with snow.

Don't allow your casualty to smoke.

Don't allow your casualty to drink alcohol.

Don't warm extremity with any **direct** heat such as a fire.

Don't burst any blisters that may form.

Don't allow thawed tissue to become frozen again.

REAL
LIFE
STORY

Frostbite while winter climbing

In the amazing winter of 2009/2010, I think many of us blew the dust off our crampons and ice axes, and headed for the white peaks of the National Parks. We'd driven up from London on the Friday, and got to our accommodation in the early hours of Saturday morning, psyched for what was to be a hard weekend, ticking off a few winter routes. A poor night's sleep and an early start did nothing to boost energy levels and, as we walked into our route, I made the mistake of keeping too many layers on and allowing myself to sweat.

On the first pitch I dropped my main gloves, leaving me with only a pair of thin nylon inners. By the time we topped out I'd got very cold, the sweat clung to my skin and the summit breeze made itself felt. We made slow but steady progress back down in the dark and straight into the pub. Buzzing from an awesome day I settled down to a pint (sensible), and a cigarette (stupid I know!). It was only then that I noticed my fingers were numb, and the finger tips were a dusky white colour. My mate peered over my shoulder and made the sort of noise that doesn't help alleviate the worry. We decided a visit to the local A&E department was probably a prudent move.

Photo: Richard Beech

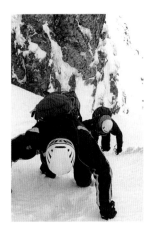

The duty doctor admitted to a lack of knowledge about cold injury, but fortunately one of the A&E nurses whose husband was a keen winter climber and had recently suffered frostbite while in the Alps, said she knew of an online UK frostbite service. So out came the mobile phone, several photos were taken of the fingers, which by this stage were turning an alarming colour of blue, and promptly ...

emailed to the UK Frostbite Advice Service, which we found through the British Mountaineering Council (BMC) website.

In the meantime the medical staff thawed my fingers in warm water and gave me some Ibuprofen. Although the docs at the A&E department were pretty sure that my fingers would slowly heal, I didn't want to take any chances, especially as I'm an IT consultant, and keyboard work is an essential part of my work. After a short discussion with my mates, we decided to drive to Coventry and let the specialists there take a look.

Many hours later we arrived in Coventry and after a brief consultation it was decided that I did need more treatment and was admitted. I think with hindsight, the frostbite was due to a range of factors apart from losing my gloves! I was tired and I'd allowed myself to get cold and worn down.

Danny Hill

Hyperthermia (too hot)

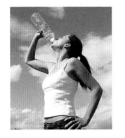

Being thirsty is a late sign of dehydration. Plan drinking stops, or use a rucksack with a drinking tube to drink while on the move. Photo: www.istockphoto.com

Adverse weather does not necessarily have to mean cold, wind, rain or snow. On occasions hot and humid weather can also cause problems. If the body is unable to get rid of excess heat produced, the core temperature starts to rise, and if left unchecked, will continue increasing until the person becomes unconscious and **dies**. Recognising the signs of heat exhaustion and heat stroke and acting promptly can save lives.

While exercising on warm days, it is sensible to consider how the body creates and loses heat, in order to anticipate and avoid any possible problems. Use common sense to reduce exercise in the hottest times of the day, remove clothing, seek shade and don't forget to replace fluids. On a particularly dry day, profuse sweating may actually go unnoticed until fluid loss is severe.

Heat exhaustion

Heat exhaustion is an increase in the core temperature; however unlike the more serious heat stroke it is less likely to cause permanent damage.

LOOK OUT FOR

Headache, nausea, dizziness and weakness. ...

Rapid pulse.

Thirst and profuse sweating.

Chills and pale skin.

Muscle cramps.

Normal or moderately raised temperature.

Other symptoms may include:

Fainting.

Vomiting.

WHAT TO DO

Cool them down:

Rest the casualty in the shade.

Place in a breeze or fan.

Remove any excess clothing.

Give the casualty plenty to drink.

Wet with cold water to increase evaporation – onto clothes or skin.

Lie the casualty down and raise the feet slightly.

Most of these casualties would probably benefit from being carefully escorted back to civilisation. Once there they should be allowed to rest and given fluids to rehydrate.

Exertional heat stroke

During heat stroke the heat regulating mechanisms of the body have become overwhelmed and can no longer cope. The body temperature starts to rise uncontrollably, creating a life-threatening emergency that requires immediate first aid treatment. The conventional description of heat stroke that occurs in the elderly and frail during heat waves is not relevant to this book; the emphasis here is on exertional heat stroke. These casualties have been exercising strenuously for a prolonged period usually in a hot environment but not always: sometimes exercising to the extreme in cooler weather can also induce exertional heat stroke. Their core temperature can become so high that major damage to the brain and vital organs is possible.

The key to treating this life-threatening condition is simple: urgently reduce the core temperature. The longer they remain hyperthermic (too hot) the more dangerous the condition.

LOOK OUT FOR

Similar to heat exhaustion but with:

Drowsiness, irritability, unsteadiness when walking.

Nausea and vomiting.

Confusion, delirium.

Rapid pulse and breathing.

Signs of shock may be present.

Dry or sweat-moistened hot skin.

May also include:

Seizures.

Shivering.

Unconscious.

WHAT TO DO

Urgently cool them down:

Remove the casualty from the heat.

Rapidly cool: wet skin and clothes, particularly in the crotch and under the arm pits.

Fan vigorously.

If conscious give them a drink.   ...

Dial 999/112 – request police – then ask for mountain rescue.

Monitor the vital signs: particularly the level of response (AVPU), as well as breathing and pulse, while you await rescue.

Be aware that rapid cooling can quickly swing the casualty towards hypothermia, and for obvious reasons this should be avoided.

It is sometimes wrongly believed that if the casualty is sweating they can't be suffering from heat stroke. On occasions the core temperature increases so quickly that the casualty is not dehydrated and the skin may still be moist with sweat.

Risk factors for hyperthermia

You are more likely to develop a heat illness if you are:

- Unfit.
- Overweight.
- Female.
- Young.
- Asthmatic.
- Diabetic.

- Pregnant.
- Heart Condition.
- Epileptic.
- Taking medication that stops sweating.
- Taking medication such as beta blockers, antidepressants, antihistamines and diuretics.

HEAT EXHAUSTION AND HEAT STROKE

Prevention is better than cure!

Wear less-insulating fabrics and encourage sweat evaporation.

Avoid exercising in high temperatures or the hottest time of day.

Drink plenty of water during exercise to keep hydrated – the best way of telling if you are hydrated is the colour of your urine. It should be clear or pale yellow. Dark yellow means you are dehydrated.

Be aware of the early signs of dehydration – headache, nausea, muscle cramps.   …

Avoid drinking alcohol and caffeine, as both increase fluid loss.

Your diet should contain enough salt to replace that being lost.

The very young and very old do not regulate their body temperature well and can become too hot very quickly.

Be aware of the risk factors that cause a person to be more prone to developing heat illnesses.

Dehydration

Dehydration means excessive loss of bodily fluid and can be a contributing factor to developing heat exhaustion and heat stroke. During exercise, humans lose fluid predominantly through sweating and less so through the action of breathing. Those exercising in heat should drink plenty before, during and after the activity; but remember it is possible to over-hydrate; drinking **too much** can be as equally dangerous. You must also be aware that even in cool temperatures it is possible to become dehydrated after strenuous exercise.

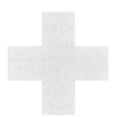

14. MOVING AND CARRYING A CASUALTY

Historically there has been a stoic attitude of self-reliance in the mountains when, if something went wrong, you had to get yourself back to civilisation by what ever means necessary. Fortunately there are now mountain rescue teams across the UK who – in an **emergency –** can be called upon to assist in giving first aid and co-ordinating an evacuation, providing the technical equipment, expertise and manpower. There should therefore no longer be any need to carry seriously injured casualties on makeshift stretchers for miles over rough terrain.

There may, however, be occasions when you might consider moving a casualty a short distance to get them away from some imminent danger (such as rockfalls, flooding, falling ice or avalanches) to find shelter or simply to enable you to start your first aid treatment. With minor injuries, or non urgent medical conditions, it may be possible to self-evacuate by physically assisting or carrying the casualty a short distance back to a road. It is important however to stress that your over-riding priority is to 'do no further harm': do not make the casualty's condition worse by moving them unnecessarily.

Safety first

Carrying a casualty, even a short distance, is often far harder than it appears. You must be realistic in your expectations of what is achievable. Practising these techniques in a non emergency situation will highlight their true limitations and the exacting toll they can place, not only on those attempting to carry or assist, but also the casualty.

Warning – as the lead first aider, it is your responsibility to ensure that nobody in your group has a pre-existing back problem, all lifts and movement are done in a controlled way and on your command. You must take charge and give clear and concise instructions throughout.

Emergency – urgent removal

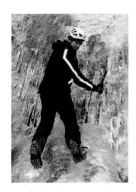

Dangers at a casualty site may include falling ice from climbers above.
Photo: Richard Beech

When a casualty is in life-threatening danger they should be removed immediately from the hazardous environment to a safer location if it is safe for you to do so. An example of this was an accident in winter involving an ice climber who fell about 50 metres, on a rope, down an ice flow sustaining tumbling injuries including a nasty arm injury. He was eventually lowered to the ground where passers-by offered their assistance. He came to rest directly underneath the ice flow, with several groups of climbers above him inadvertently knocking off huge chunks of ice. The first aider decided it was too dangerous to stay there and with a little help from others around, moved him 30 feet or so clear of the hazard and onto safer ground.

If the casualty is conscious they may be able to assist in their move such as placing an arm around your shoulder or shuffling along the ground. If they are unconscious or unable to assist, you may simply have to drag them clear of the danger, or if there are others around, perform a quick grab and carry.

The biggest concern most first aiders express is "but what if the casualty has a spinal injury?" Your priority should always be their removal from the danger; however it is possible to do this while being mindful of a potential spinal injury which will be discussed later.

All techniques to carry or move a casualty mentioned in this chapter can be used in the urgent situation.

Non emergency

Moving a casualty in a non-emergency situation needs to be done after careful thought and consideration. Their injuries or medical condition may make any movement impossible or even dangerous. The weight and size of the casualty is important; always evaluate the load and be realistic about whether the casualty is too heavy. Consider the number and fitness of the available helpers and evaluate the terrain you are thinking of crossing or moving over.

Check to see if there is any equipment around that could be improvised to assist in the move such as walking poles, ropes, survival bag, or a group shelter. Another point to consider – which is sometimes lost in the enthusiasm of wanting to 'have a go' – is the casualty's comfort; what may appear straightforward to the carriers may actually be quite unpleasant for the casualty. If they feel uneasy about your proposed method of carrying, they may become increasingly anxious which will only serve to intensify their pain and distress.

With a non-emergency situation – where there is no urgency – plan your move thoroughly and have everything you need in place beforehand, such as insulating the ground where you intend to move to. If possible avoid the need to move the casualty more than once.

Principles and guidelines

Generally speaking a casualty should be treated in the position you find them and only moved for a good reason before making your assessment. An example of this would be a casualty who has leapt over a mountain stream, broken their ankle and then landed in the stream. It might be prudent for you to support the injured ankle and have them carefully inch their way back onto dry land **before** you start your treatment.

Similarly if – during cold, wet, windy weather conditions – a shelter can be quickly reached (such as a nearby tent or mountain bothy) without harm to the casualty, then this may be a more suitable environment in which to carry out your assessment and any necessary treatment.

Assisting a walking casualty

With a casualty who is able and willing to walk, it may be possible for you to assist them. Offering a steady hand and a few words of encouragement can sometimes enable the casualty to make slow but steady progress.

Monitor the walking casualty carefully. Be prepared to alter your descent route to accommodate any limitations in movement that the injury may inflict. Be aware that a casualty with an arm sling will experience issues with balance.

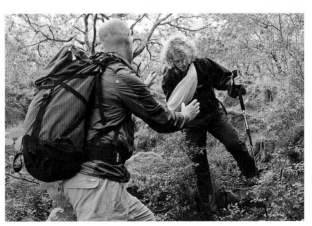

If walking poles are available they can be utilised to give the casualty a little more support and aid in balancing. Another simple technique is to place someone to the side of the casualty who can be used as support. If the terrain allows, use two people (one on either side), with the casualty's arms around their shoulders. The assisted walking casualty will need close monitoring and if necessary you should be prepared to re-evaluate your plan; you may have to convert this into some form of carry, or even call for mountain rescue.

Carrying a casualty

If the casualty is unable to walk, but capable of holding themselves upright, it might be worth considering an improvised carry. If they are unable to support themselves upright you may wish to consider an improvised stretcher carry. Think carefully about the size of your casualty and the number and fitness of those offering to help. Use your common sense. With all carrying techniques it is important to monitor the casualty (and those carrying) and be prepared to re-assess the situation; call for help if required. The following are a selection of carrying techniques used in the remote environment.

One person carry

RUCKSACK CARRY

Turn the rucksack upside down and ask the casualty to step into the loops created by the shoulder straps. Pull the rucksack up high until the shoulder straps of the rucksack are in the groin. The carrier then bends down and feeds the rucksack straps onto their shoulders. If available place padding on the top of the carrier's shoulders underneath the straps.

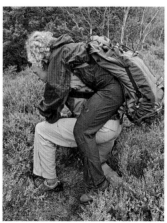
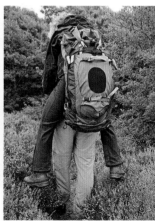

ONE PERSON SPLIT ROPE CARRY

Carrying someone with a rope is actually fairly comfortable for the carrier (depending on the size of the casualty) and is easy to adjust to different heights by simply re-coiling the rope making the loops shorter or longer. Ensure the knot in the rope is high enough up the casualty's back to prevent them from falling out backwards. If available pad underneath the rope that lies over the carrier's shoulders. At the front use a sling or belt to bring the coils of rope together.

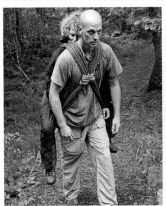 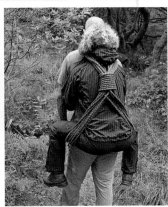

Two person carry

TWO PERSON SPLIT ROPE CARRY

As with the one person technique the split rope is easily adjusted to suit the height of the casualty by re-coiling the rope making the loops shorter or longer. Place extra padding – such as a spare fleece or jacket – over the knot to provide added casualty comfort. Ideally the carrier's should be of a similar height. If available place extra padding under the rope that lies on the carrier's shoulders.

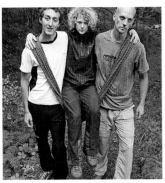 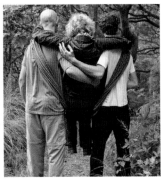

RUCKSACKS WITH WALKING POLES CARRY

Measure the distance from the outer edge of one rucksack to outer edge of the other (include the casualty). Extend the poles to that length then tape together. Stand the carriers side by side and feed the walking poles through the gap at the base of the rucksack just above the waist belt. If extra padding is available place this over the poles. Use as many poles as are available and is comfortable.

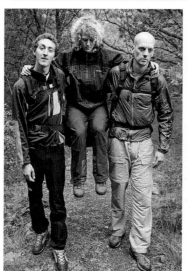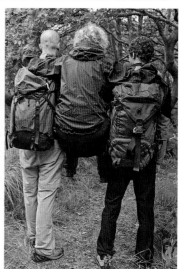

Improvised stretchers

Stretchers can be improvised from any sheeted material such as an orange survival bag, tent or group shelter. A stretcher carry takes a considerable number of people and all injuries must be treated and immobilised before transfer. **Do not** move a suspected spinal injury (including head injuries), pelvic or thigh bone fractures – or anyone suffering from shock – on an improvised stretcher.

As the lead first aider, you will be expected to take control and clearly brief your helpers on all aspects of the move. Make sure the group know where they are moving to and that all moves are done on your command.

Guidance on lifting and carrying

1. With the conscious casualty always inform them of what you are about to do. Monitor the casualty by talking to them.

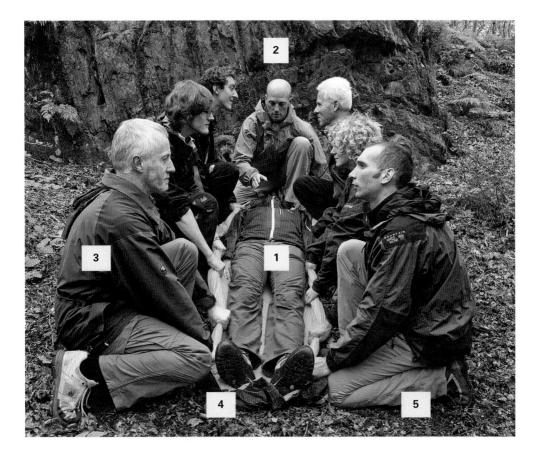

2. The lead first aider should take the position at the head. The lift, move and lower are done on their command.

3. When lifting, keep the back straight and eyes looking straight ahead.

4. Position yourself as close to the casualty as possible. Use the strong muscles of the thighs and buttocks to lift.

5. Adopt a stable base with your feet shoulder width apart and avoid twisting your back; if you need to pivot use your feet.

Think carefully about your route before you decide on a stretcher carry. A footpath needs to be wide enough to take not only the width of the stretcher, but the carriers on both sides. Also consider the gradient of your route; a steep slope with a casualty that is not secured to the stretcher is a recipe for disaster. If you have sufficient people, ask one person to lead in front to warn the carriers of oncoming obstacles, or changes in terrain such as a rock step, loose scree, etc.

SHEET STRETCHER

As the lead first aider you take control of the head. Place your helpers down either side. The heaviest part of the casualty are the shoulders and upper chest, therefore place the stronger carriers there.

There are a number of ways to lift this type of stretcher. Some people place stones down the side of the orange survival bag and hold onto them, others feed walking poles down the edges and use them to gain purchase. The technique shown here is simply to roll the bag tightly towards the casualty.

The lift and lower must be on the lead first aider's command. Ensure all helpers have been briefed clearly on what is expected.

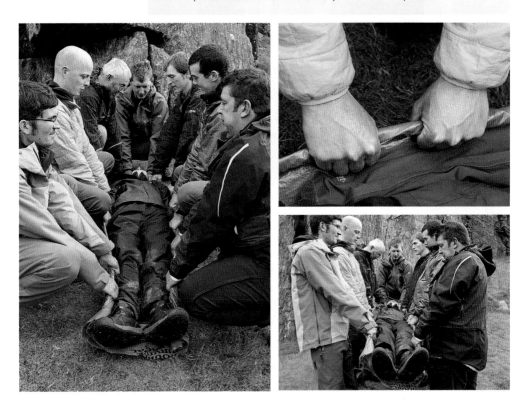

If conscious casualties may be able to move themselves onto the sheet for the carry, or you may have to assist them. If they are unconscious you will need to gently roll them onto it.

ROLLING THE UNCONSCIOUS CASUALTY ONTO A SHEET

Roll the sheet length ways, leaving a short section unrolled. Place the rolled section next to the unconscious casualty and tuck under the nearest arm and leg.

Bring the casualty over into a safe airway position onto the sheet.

Pull the surplus rolled section outwards.

If not intending to stretcher the casualty, this technique can be used to help insulate them by bringing the surplus edge of the sheet back over to cover them.

Gently turn the casualty onto their back in the middle of the sheet.

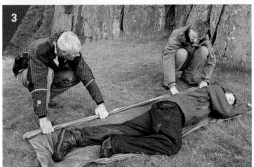

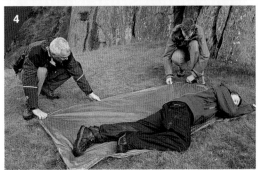

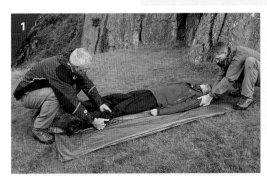

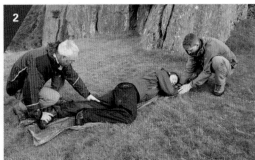

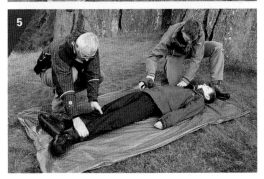

WALKING POLES AND JACKET STRETCHER

*This stretcher should **not** be used with spinal injury casualties..*

Take 3 jackets, turn the sleeves inside out and zip them up. Take two sets of walking poles and duct tape them together at the bottom ends. Lay the jackets on the floor and feed the poles down through the inverted sleeves. Carriers take hold of the poles to lift.

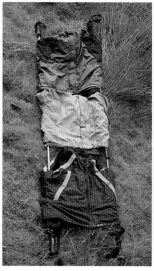
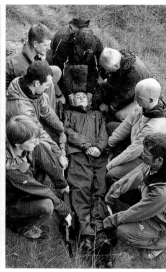
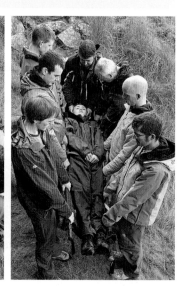

Moving a spinal injury casualty

Move this casualty the shortest distance necessary until safety can be reached.

There are few times when you should consider moving a spinal casualty; however danger is certainly one of them. If there are a number of people available you might be able to organise a spinal lift and carry. Hold the head in a neutral position and during the lift and carry aim to keep the whole of the spine, including the neck and head, in a straight line and try to avoid any bending or twisting of their back or neck.

SPINAL LIFT AND CARRY

Hold the head in a neutral position. The carriers crouch along either side of the casualty. They take hold of the clothing just underneath the casualty and pull tightly towards them. Carriers at the legs slide their hands underneath both legs.

On your command initiate the lift keeping the casualty as straight as possible. Give clear instructions.   ...

Once standing, move slowly in the direction of planned travel. Keep the spine, head and neck in as straight a line as possible. If the casualty is conscious, ask them to keep their arms crossed over their chest.

When you have reached your destination, stop the group and lower the casualty on your command. Keep the spine, head and neck as straight as possible.

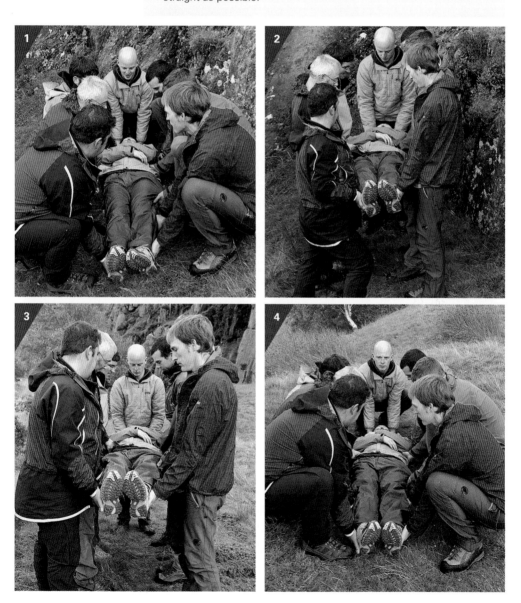

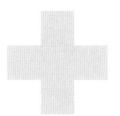

15. WORKING WITH RESCUE SERVICES

While taking part in outdoor activities it is inevitable that on occasions people will become injured or simply feel unwell. In an ideal situation you will be able to offer some level of first aid and then evacuate the casualty yourself. However sometimes the incident will be beyond your basic first aid skills or perhaps you are simply unable to self-evacuate. In these situations you will need help from a local mountain rescue team, who in turn may use search dogs to locate you and perhaps deploy a helicopter to assist in the rescue. An understanding of how these emergency services work will make the whole rescue process run more efficiently and safely for all concerned.

Calling for mountain rescue

Group/Emergency shelter: this mobile shelter provides an excellent escape from the elements and crucially packs down small.

Once you stop moving, the casualty and everyone else in the party will in all probability start to become cold; if you are not adequately prepared, hypothermia may become an additional problem. Having decided to call for help try to insulate yourself and the casualty from the ground and provide some form of shelter, such as a group shelter (also known as a kisu, bothy bag or emergency shelter).

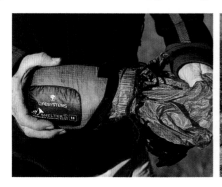

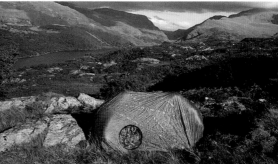

Your next task is to gather information to pass on to the rescue services.

WHAT TO DO

Make a note of the following:

What has happened (in detail), and when.

Name, sex, and age of casualty.

Nature of the injuries or illness, any medical conditions, are they taking any medication?

The number in the group, their ages and any medical conditions they may have?

A description of clothing and colour are essential.

Grid reference of your location.

Weather conditons can be useful, for example in or out of cloud.

Summoning help

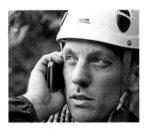

Once you have gathered this information you will need to summon help. Mountain rescue teams come under the control of the police therefore you must dial 999/112, request **POLICE**, then ask for **MOUNTAIN RESCUE**. The police operators are trained initially to take down **your** name, age, date of birth and address before they ask you about your incident; be prepared to give these details. When they have all the necessary information, they will alert the nearest mountain rescue team.

GETTING HELP IN THE UK MOUNTAINS

Mobile phone – Dial 999/112. If registered with the EmergencySMS text service you may be able to send a text.

Telephone – Dial 999/112. Using a landline will mean someone has to leave the casualty and return to a road head or a remote house.

Shouting – Make sure you shout 'help' so that passersby know you require assistance.

International distress signal – 6 blasts of a whistle or 6 flashes of a torch repeated every minute (if replying to this request for help, respond with 3 blasts or 3 flashes, repeated every minute). Keep signalling even if someone replies. ...

Morse Code SOS – 3 short, 3 long, 3 short ($\cdot \cdot \cdot$ – – – $\cdot \cdot \cdot$) blasts of a whistle or flashes of a torch every minute (if replying, respond with 3 blasts or 3 flashes, repeated every minute). Keep signalling even if someone replies.

EMERGENCY SMS TEXT SERVICE TO 999

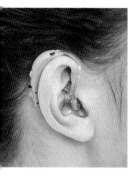

EmergencySMS is a national UK service enabling deaf, hard of hearing or speech impaired individuals to text their emergency to 999. The service is available to anyone in the UK whether they are hearing impaired or not.

You must register your phone before you can use the service.

Text the word 'register' to 999.

Photo:
www.istockphoto.com

You will then receive text messages about the service.

When you have read the messages reply by texting 'yes' to 999.

You will then receive a text message telling you that your mobile phone is registered or if there is a problem with your registration.

For further information visit www.emergencysms.org.uk

Some general considerations

Once you have dialled 999/112 stay off your phone so that the rescue services can contact you.

If using a mobile phone, give a lead mobile number and a reserve in case the battery runs out. Be aware that there will be a time delay between your calling for help and the rescue team contacting you.

If visibility is poor or you are off the beaten track, it may be useful to use a rope (if available) laid out on the ground to guide rescuers to your position.

Working with mountain rescue

The vast majority of mountain rescue bases are unmanned; this means that it is unlikely there are a group of people sitting around waiting for your emergency. As unpaid volunteers, the majority of rescue team members are going about their daily routine; you must expect a time delay between your call and their response.

The reason for this delay can be better appreciated when you consider what is involved in a 'call out'. Although the following sequence of events is specific to the Llanberis Mountain Rescue Team, there will be a similar set of procedures for every UK rescue team.

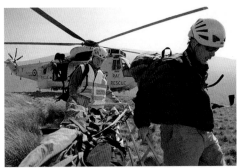

Mountain Rescue Team members being deployed onto the mountain by RAF Sea King helicopter.
Photo: Mark Reeves

After your 999/112 call to the police, a pager and SMS text message is sent to all team members notifying them that someone has dialled 999/112 and is requesting assistance. One of the designated volunteer co-ordinators will stop what they are doing and phone 'police control' to collect the information given to the police in the initial emergency call. If the initial information from the police is life-threatening, the co-ordinator will page/SMS the team to go immediately to the mountain rescue base; they will then attempt to call the informant back to let them know the rescue team has been called out, whether a helicopter has been requested and if so, its expected time of arrival.

Alternatively, if the incident is not life-threatening, the co-ordinator will page/SMS text the team to let them know they are investigating and request the team to go on 'stand by'. The co-ordinator will then attempt to call the informant back in order to gather more information before summoning the team to a call out. Remember, if you have dialled 999/112 from a mobile phone that only allows emergency calls, the rescue services will be unable to call you back. It is important, therefore, that you give as much detail as possible to the police in your initial phone call.

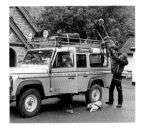

Loading rescue equipment onto the vehicle roof ready for deployment.
Photo: Howard Wilkinson

When team members arrive at the mountain rescue base, they are briefed on the incident and allocated tasks. Equipment is gathered, signed out, team vehicles mobilised, rescuers placed into groups then eventually sent out on the rescue.

It will, in all likelihood, take the rescue team as long to get to where you are as it did for you to get there! This means you may be left with your casualty for some considerable time. It is easy to feel abandoned and forgotten during this stage – but be patient.

When the rescue team arrives they will need to establish exactly what happened and the nature of the injury or illness; be prepared to give this information and if you have completed a **casualty report form** hand this over. You may be asked to assist, given a specific task, or simply instructed to remain out of the way. This can sometimes be a very busy, confusing and intense time, so try to listen to the instructions and be as helpful as you can.

Photo: Brian Wills

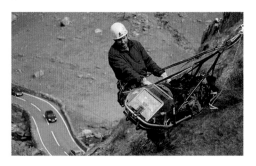

REAL
LIFE
STORY

Climbing accident

Looking at his feet I could see the left one was broken straight away. I grabbed my mobile and rang 999, asking for police and then mountain rescue. I feel grateful, every day since, that I knew not to get an ambulance, as even though we weren't far from a track; he needed to be carried over some difficult terrain. What would I have done if there was no signal? Would I have stayed with Steve and sent someone else off to phone?

It's confusing when you ring up because you get put through to the police control room, so they say "police". I said, "I need mountain rescue, there is a young man fallen off a climb, definitely broken ankle possibly two, and I am not sure about his back, although he is moving around". As I said that I realised that he shouldn't be moving around. The woman said she would get hold of mountain rescue and call me back, to stay where I was in signal, and she asked about my battery life (not good, why hadn't I charged it!). I described where we were; I didn't know the grid reference; we were climbing, so I gave the route name!

I remembered the ABCs of first aid, and could see that he was breathing ok, although sobbing in pain. I tried to keep him still but he wasn't having any of it. I asked the others for some coats to keep him warm, but he just pushed them off.

After a while (it seemed like ages), the police rang back, took some more details, and said that mountain rescue would be calling me soon. This next bit seemed to go on forever. I would have welcomed anyone who could tell me what to do at that point, but the other people around seemed to be looking to me for what to do.   ...

Finally mountain rescue called back and I was so relieved to hear a reassuring voice. They took some more details and then said that the team and a helicopter were already on their way, and to keep Steve still.

I think it was probably only half an hour or so before the team arrived, and they all looked cool, calm and collected. They were very slick, working together really well. I was worried about being in the way but no-one asked me to move. I kept holding Steve's hand, and he just kept looking at me. Instantly, the rescue team had a good rapport with him asking questions, the odd joke, getting him comfortable, relaying information, so the person at the head end was the only one Steve had to focus on. I thought that was really important, because suddenly there were a lot of people around and it was confusing. They checked him over everywhere, and were reassuring and gentle. It was good to be involved in things; it gave me something to do.

When Steve was on the stretcher and ready to go up in the helicopter, they carried him off around the corner and I didn't follow. I wanted to stay out of the way and let them do their job. Immediately after he had gone, someone asked if I was ok. At that point I felt tears well up, I think I said "no" then burst into tears.

Rebecca Williams

Working with search dogs

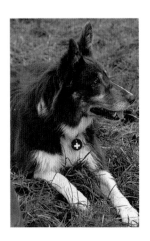

If you call for help but don't know where you are, it is possible search dogs as well as rescue team members will be called out to assist. Search dogs are trained to pick up human scent carried by the wind. Once a dog picks up your scent it will run directly to you. It is then trained to return to its handler and indicate that it has found something, usually by barking. The dog will then continue to shuttle between you and its handler, until the dog, you and the handler are all together.

It is important if you have called for help to stay where you are; do not wander around. The dog is trained to ignore moving people, and other loose dogs, so the best advice is to stay put. If you have a dog with you, tie it up. If a search dog finds you, do not grab hold of it or attempt to give it food; allow it to return to its handler to indicate it has found you.

It takes about 2–3 years to train a search dog and its handler before they are ready to be placed on the 'Call Out' list. The whole emphasis on search dog training revolves around repetition, fun and a reward for 'finding'. Photo: Rohan Holt

Working with helicopters

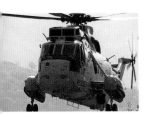

Helicopters are sometimes used in conjunction with mountain rescues, although this will depend on the seriousness of your situation, weather conditions and the availability of the aircraft. If mountain rescue request a helicopter, it may be with you long before the rescue team itself; you should therefore be familiar with some basic procedures to keep everyone safe and help the aircraft find you.

Once the helicopter has spotted you, a crew member may fire a smoke canister close to your location. When it hits the ground it will send off bright orange/red smoke which will indicate the wind direction. Leave the canister alone, it will be very hot! Photo: Rob Booth

The vast majority of helicopter rescues that take place in UK Mountains are done by Royal Air Force and Royal Navy Sea King helicopters. There are however occasions when rescue teams may use other helicopters belonging to other agencies such as the Coastguard or Air Ambulance. Not all of these aircraft types are able to winch, as a result they may have to find somewhere flat to land and the crew will make their way to you on foot.

Regardless of which helicopter attends you will need to attract their attention. A description of your clothing – particularly the colours – is essential. It is not uncommon for the casualty and their group to be wearing dark colours, making them totally camouflaged. This can make locating them from the air at best challenging, at worst impossible.

Things you need to do

Make it known that you need help! That might sound obvious but on a busy mountainside it may actually be quite difficult to work out who needs assistance.

Day: If possible open up and pin out an orange survival bag on the ground; from the air this is very visible. Alternatively stand in a Y position with your feet together and your arms open wide above your head.

When you see the helicopter approaching stand in a Y shape, as shown here: preferably with your back to the wind. This tells the aircraft that it is you who needs assistance.

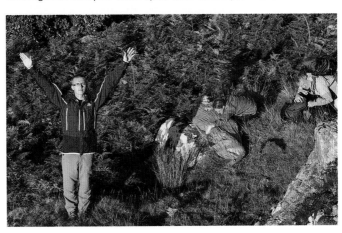

Night: Shine your torch directly onto the floor, or use a sweeping motion on the ground. Alternatively use a light stick on a string spun around your head. If you are caught out with no torch, the back light on a mobile phone can be useful for attracting attention, or the flash on a camera, even the light from an iPod.

LIGHT STICKS USED TO DRAW ATTENTION

Someone holding a light stick at night appears quite small. Compare that to the effect of spinning the light stick on string.

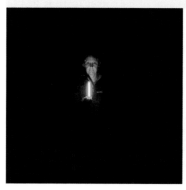 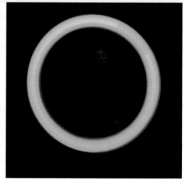

Try to control bystanders by asking them to stay at least 50 metres away; the down draught on a helicopter can be immense and it is possible to be swept off your feet. For this reason it is advisable to secure any loose clothing or equipment and as the aircraft approaches, kneel or sit down. If you are winched on board the aircraft listen very carefully to the crew and do exactly what they say.

HELICOPTER DON'TS

Don't just wave at the helicopter, everybody waves!

Don't approach the helicopter under any circumstances, let the crew members come to you.

Don't try to assist the winchman in his task, allow him to make his own way to you.

Don't shine your head torch directly at the aircraft, at night this destroys the night vision of the crew, which may seriously hamper any rescue attempt.

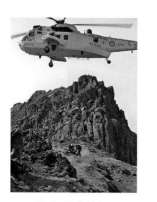

Photo: Craig Holt

Unlike many other countries, the use of the military search and rescue helicopters in civilian rescues is currently free of charge to those being rescued. These helicopters however, are responsible for vast areas including maritime regions; therefore the rescue team co-ordinating will give careful consideration before using such a valuable asset.

Fallen climber

REAL
LIFE
STORY

At last the RAF helicopter arrived. It hovered for a while, and the down blast was startling. There was a pair of climbers sitting at the top of the incline. I'd stopped them from entering the area of the accident and they were now sitting almost directly under the helicopter, clinging to their lunches and rucksacks. I frantically waved at them to go away, and eventually they got the message. I glanced towards the group huddled around the casualty, trying to protect her from the helicopter down blast. Empty rucksacks, items of clothing, climbing shoes and plastic bags were all flying about. A helmet and a chalk bag bounced like tumble weed over an edge, and down to another level of the quarry.

The helicopter rose slightly and I thought it was going to move away. As it climbed, the pilot must have spotted the casualty and a paramedic (winchman), was lowered down. He made his way to the group and immediately set about his assessment of the casualty. I returned to my viewpoint to direct members of the mountain rescue team who were coming up on foot. Minutes later, three arrived in quick succession. Help had taken about an hour after I made the first call.

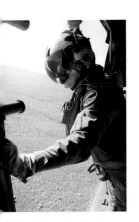

RAF winchman in the door
of a Sea King helicopter.
Photo: Mark Reeves

Together they worked at assessing the many injuries and how best to treat them. The casualty's harness was cut off and a broken pelvis was suspected. One person was holding her head still and the rest of us did our best to help where we could. Loose items were gathered up and rocks placed on them.

When the casualty was on the stretcher, I moved back to help. Jobs were delegated and commands given to ensure we worked together. I had the job of holding the oxygen mask over her nose as she was carried towards the helicopter. This had returned and landed on a small, uneven platform surrounded by vertical rock and steep slopes. I did my best to hold the mask in position, without pushing it against her injured face, as I stumbled through the deafening noise and wind blasting down upon us. We arrived at the helicopter and passed her up. We were moved away from the helicopter then up a small slope and stayed there while the helicopter took off.

Storm Bate

Calls for help in the UK Mountains for first aid reasons will never be questioned. However, it must be remembered that Mountain Rescue teams and Search and Rescue Dog Associations are run by volunteers who give of their time freely. They exist to provide an **emergency service**.

A sight you will hopefully
never see!
Photo: Elidir Owen

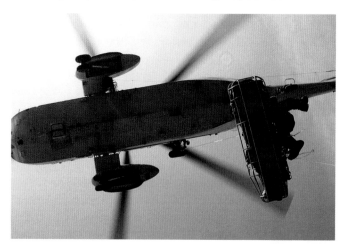

16. OUTDOOR FIRST AID KITS

People often ask what they should carry in their first aid kit – and the standard answer is "well that depends". It depends on a number of things, specifically the activity being undertaken, the number of people involved and your level of first aid training. A mountain biking first aid kit taken on a day out with a friend may look very different from a first aid kit put together to lead a group of walkers in the mountains.

I questioned 200 people who either worked or played in the outdoors about what they carried in their remote first aid kit. Although there is a consensus of certain first aid items, no two people carried the same type and number of things in the same container (unless they used the same first aid kit). Even those who indicated they carried a shop-bought first aid kit appeared to personalise its contents. It is impossible to advocate a 'standard' outdoor first aid kit. However, I can highlight some of the issues to consider when assembling your own kit.

Container

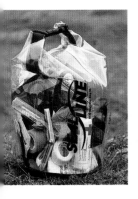

My research indicated that 53% of the sample chose to put their kit into a 'dry bag' (a watertight bag that seals), with 32% opting for a shop-bought first aid kit and 13% a plastic container of some kind. Keeping the shop-bought first aid kit dry appeared to be an issue, with a number of people placing it inside a dry bag. The other 2% used random containers included zip pouches, plastic bags, a military first aid kit bag and a tin box.

Dry bags are made from plastic (some are completely transparent), fabric coated with plastic, or waterproof fabric. The top of the bag is folded down several times and fastened with a clip.

Some of the shop-bought kits have handy little compartments to divide items into organised sections; dry bags on the other hand do not. This can be overcome by grouping items together and packing them into waterproof storage bags such as those produced by Aloksak.

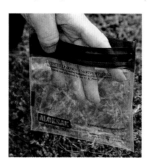

Aloksak waterproof storage bags. These handy transparent bags are waterproof down to sixty metres and come in a variety of sizes.

Contents

The following list shows all first aid items that 10% or more of the 200 individuals questioned included in their first aid kits.

Examination gloves	95%	Casualty report form	48%
Medical tape	93%	Gauze swabs	42%
Support bandage (e.g. crepe)	92%	Aspirin (for heart attacks)	36%
Scissors	91%	Saline	36%
Triangular bandage	90%	Eye bandage	35%
Plasters	88%	Antihistamine tablets	34%
Wound dressing	87%	Glucose	33%
Medi Wipes	81%	Rehydration sachet/tablets	33%
Non/low adherent dressing	80%	Catastrophic bleed dressing	32%
Painkiller medication	74%	Clinical waste bags	32%
Safety pins	72%	Burns dressing	32%
Wound closure strips	67%	Disinfectant	26%
Blister plasters	67%	Splint	23%
Face shield	64%	Tick tweezers	14%
Tweezers	59%	Notebook	10%
Duct tape	48%		

First aid kit core elements

When putting together an outdoor first aid kit there has to be compromise; you can't take everything 'just in case'. Your aim should be to do as much as you can with as little as possible and consider improvising where necessary. Another top tip is to purchase good quality products that can endure being stuffed into the bottom of rucksacks, or forced into pockets.

The vast majority of those people questioned (80%) appear to carry a **core** of first aid items, to which they then add their own personal preferences. The core kit identified contains the following items.

Examination gloves (95%)

Every first aid kit should contain examination gloves. Of those respondents who identified which type of gloves they carried, 32% said nitrile, 21% latex, and 18% vinyl. Interestingly, a number of those who carried latex gloves also carried another type of glove, possibly in case they came across a casualty who was allergic to latex. Be aware of this if you currently only carry latex gloves!

Tape (93%)

Tape is a useful multipurpose item and many people carry a number of different types. Medical tapes include Micropore (62%), Zinc Oxide (38%) and Transpore (1%). My research indicates that in the outdoors Transpore appears to be the most versatile general purpose tape, it is a transparent, breathable hypoallergenic plastic tape which has strong adhesion. Other non-medical tapes carried included duct tape (48%) and insulation tape (3%).

Support bandage (92%)

Support bandages included elastic adhesive or crepe. Elastic adhesive bandages are designed specifically for support of soft tissue injuries, such as a sprained ankle. A crepe bandage however is multifunctional and may also be used to secure dressings in place and, if wide enough, as a tie to help immobilise fractures.

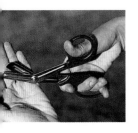

Tuff cut scissors. These scissors are designed with a small bar at the bottom to help them glide along the skin.

Scissors (91%)

Many people carry scissors on a multi tool (or a pen knife), which they may carry for a different purpose. Others carry medical scissors which can be used to cut tape, dressings to size, or clothing to access an injured area. Be cautious about cutting people's clothes off, it is not something you should routinely do! However, if it allows you to access an injury in order to dress a wound make sure the scissors you use do not accidentally cut the skin.

Triangular bandage (90%)

Triangular bandages continue to be a popular addition to most first aid kits. If you are going to carry this type of bandage, buy a decent quality cotton one. Remember, as long as it doesn't get covered in blood you can always wash it and use it again.

Plasters (88%)

These can be bought separately or in a strip. Once again buy good quality plasters and keep them dry and clean. A very popular plaster for use in the outdoors appears to be Nexcare, produced by 3M. The tape is incredibly sticky (it will even stick to damp skin) and stays put. You can buy a water-proof version and they are latex-free and hypoallergenic.

Wound dressing (87%)

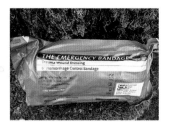

This is a dressing pad attached to a bandage and sealed in a plastic wrapper which come in a variety of sizes. They are not designed to deal with a catastrophic bleed and so will only manage moderate amounts of leakage. A compromise to cover all eventualities would be to carry a modern military dressing, such as **The emergency bandage: trauma wound dressing** (also known as an Israeli bandage or dressing), which is designed to stop all types of bleeds from minor to life-threatening.

Photo: Katherine Wills

Medi wipes (81%)

These are handy little pre-packed moist medical wipes. They can be used to clean wounds and if necessary sterilise equipment such as scissors or a needle.

Non and low adherent dressings (80%)

These are thin dressing pads, which are secured in place with tape, or a bandage, and used to stem fairly light to moderate leakage. If you carry the larger size, you can always cut it down to dress a smaller wound.

Group shelter

Any good wilderness survival course will teach you that the first principle of surviving in the outdoors is protection from the elements. For this reason, I would suggest that at the core of any good outdoor first aid kit should be some means of creating a shelter. The easiest way to achieve this is to carry a group shelter: a big windproof bag which resembles the outside of a tent and allows people to gather underneath to shelter from the elements (also known as a kisu, bothy bag or emergency shelter). This shelter can be put up anywhere and will protect you, and others, from the wind, rain, sleet or snow. They are great for lunch stops in bad weather, but crucially they form a vital piece of kit for managing a first aid incident in the outdoors.

Other useful items

There are many items on the list which you may wish to add to this core first aid kit depending on the activity chosen. Those venturing into areas where ticks live may wish to add tick tweezers, and if planning a wilderness camp it might be sensible to carry burn dressings. If you work in an outdoor centre and the clients are using centre boots, it may be wise to add blister plasters. The list is endless. However there are a number of items worthy of further discussion.

Medications

A significant number of people questioned (74%) carry some kind of over the counter painkiller; including paracetamol, ibuprofen, co-codamol (para-cetamol plus codeine) and co-dydramol (paracetamol plus dihydrocodeine). A number of other drugs are also being carried, including aspirin for heart attacks (36%), oral antihistamines (34%), asthma inhalers (8%), tablets for diarrhoea (3%) and decongestants (2%).

Where medication is concerned, first aiders need to act thoughtfully, appropriately and with a huge dose of common sense. If you can purchase a medication over the counter then that medication can and should be used in a responsible way. Offering drugs to a casualty empowers them to make their own decision, but gaining consent is paramount. Those who work in the outdoors under an umbrella organisation, such as a local education authority, may find restrictions as to what they can and can not carry in their first aid kit; this may also include medication. You need to be aware of any restrictions placed on you by your workplace and operate within these boundaries.

If you choose to carry over-the-counter medications in your outdoor first aid kit, it would be advisable to copy the dosage and all contraindications (circumstances when a certain drug should not be taken) onto waterproof paper and store this with the medication in your kit. Note that some common medications – such as asthma inhalers – are a prescription-only drug.

Glucose (33%)

Some form of glucose (gels or tablets) is carried by 33% of those sampled. Glucose is a simple sugar and serves as the main source of energy in the body. There are a number of conditions you can treat with glucose including hypoglycaemia (low blood sugar), hypothermia (too cold) and exhaustion.

Clinical waste bags (32%)

Once you have finished dressing any wounds it is useful to have something you can place any rubbish into. This does not have to be the yellow clinical waste bags you see in hospitals; a simple sandwich bag or nappy sack will suffice, to hold things like used medical wipes or anything contaminated with blood. Some people improvise and use their examination gloves; after treating the casualty they grab the waste in their gloved hand, then peel the examination glove off turning it inside out around the waste and finish by tying a knot in the top.

Casualty report form (46%)

A casualty report form contains a set of guidance notes to help you gather relevant and appropriate information for the rescue services, as well as helping you to assess your casualty and monitor their vital signs whilst awaiting rescue. There are many different types of casualty report forms and an example of one is presented here. The most effective way of using this form in the outdoors is to print it onto waterproof paper and carry a pencil to write with. If you laminate the form, use a chinagraph pencil; permanent pens on laminate in the rain do not work.

Download this casualty report form from www.activefirstaid.co.uk/CasualtyReportForm.pdf

The casualty report form should remain with the casualty at all times and be handed over to the rescue services on their arrival.

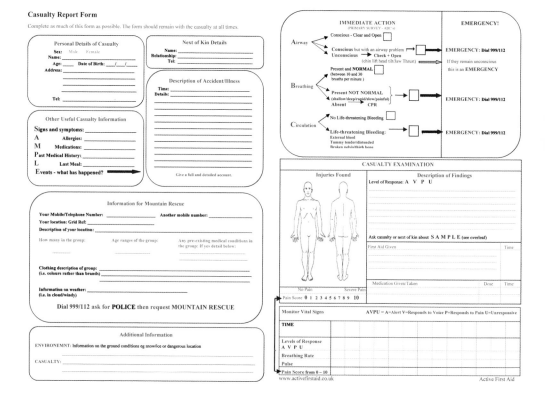

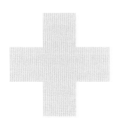

17. POST TRAUMATIC STRESS DISORDER

When we tie the laces of our rock boots, pack our wing for a day's paragliding, or get our rucksack out of the car and start the day's adventure, few of us expect things to go wrong. Sometimes we experience unplanned adventures and near misses which may rattle us briefly, but makes for a fantastic story with the occasional embellishment thrown in for good measure. But sometimes events unravel and cause the rug to be pulled from under us. This experience can be overwhelming and difficult to deal with.

Photo:
www.istockphoto.com

By their nature, accidents in the mountains have the potential to be very distressing, not only for the casualty but also for the family and friends of those involved, people who witness the event, or those called upon to offer assistance.

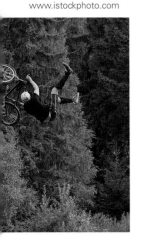

A TRAUMATIC EXPERIENCE

A traumatic experience is one in which there has been a serious threat to your life, or threat or harm to your children, partner, close relative or friend. It could be witnessing another person, someone you don't know, being injured, or killed. The event doesn't have to actually be life-threatening; it just has to be seen that way. Your response to that event would have involved a feeling of horror, fear or helplessness.

After an incident

Immediately after a traumatic event, people are often stunned and numb. Some appear to become 'cut off' from the real world and from what's going on around them. It may be difficult to accept the traumatic event has happened and for some they even behave as though it hasn't. This can be misinterpreted as either being 'strong' and dealing with it, or simply not caring. Each person's reaction to a traumatic event is different; it will depend on how they make sense of the event and its potential consequences. Reactions may include, crying, hysteria, being utterly devastated, grief stricken and unable to cope. Being upset is a natural human emotion: it is quite normal.

Post trauma reaction

In the first few weeks following a traumatic event it is not unusual to be particularly tearful and sad, feel lethargic, struggle to concentrate on the simplest of things and become easily distracted. For most, there is a period of coming to terms with what happened, and then the stress symptoms start to disappear. However, not everyone is so lucky, and for some the process just gets stuck. What started off as a normal stress response becomes a long term problem – this is post traumatic stress disorder (PTSD).

How it might affect you

If you've been involved in, or had to deal with the aftermath of, an accident (or simply been witness to it) then you are almost certainly going to be affected in some way by the experience. Symptoms usually develop immediately after the incident; however for some these can be delayed for weeks, months or even years.

Flashbacks and nightmares

One of the most distressing symptoms of post-traumatic stress is the reliving of the event. During the day these can take the form of 'flashbacks', in which you relive the incident to such an extent that it feels like it is happening all over again. Some people also experience 'intrusions'; when images of the event just randomly pop into your mind. Flashbacks and intrusions can be triggered by such things as smells or sounds which you link to the event; these can last from a split second to several minutes.

At night you may have difficulty sleeping and any sleep you are able to get can be invaded by distressing dreams and nightmares of the event. Both flashbacks and nightmares can seem incredibly real: not only do they invade your mind, but you can feel the emotions and the physical sensations, such as sounds, smells, fear and the grief of the event. These constant invasions can become distressing, adding fuel to the mistaken belief that you are 'going mad'.

Avoidance

To cope with the flashbacks and nightmares you may start to avoid places, situations or people which remind you of the traumatic event. Another common avoidance technique is not wishing to talk about what happened. You begin to communicate less with people, and may become emotionally withdrawn and depressed.

Hyper arousal

Hyper arousal feels as if you are constantly in a state of 'red alert'; anxious and on the edge. This is the body's adrenaline-led fight-or-flight response and results in physical reactions such as increased heart rate and breathing, and sweaty palms. This rush of adrenaline is responsible for two of the most common behaviours seen in post-traumatic stress; irritability and anger. This is the 'fight' part of the response which (when there is actually no threat) is directed towards anything or anyone around you, even your loved ones.

The state of hyper arousal leads some people to experience panic attacks, which may strike at any time and be quite debilitating. As the attacks increase you might start to avoid places where they happen; for some this leads to becoming completely housebound. Sleep problems are also made worse by the constant fight-or-flight response; you may experience difficulties in getting off to sleep as well as waking very early.

Other symptoms of PTSD

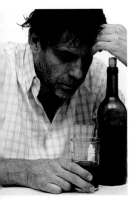

Apart from the reactions already mentioned, a whole host of other physical symptoms may accompany PTSD. In fact, it may be in the pursuance of getting answers to the physical aches and pains which direct the medical profession to the diagnosis and treatment of PTSD. These can include stomach upsets, diarrhoea, heartburn, chest pains, tremors, feeling very cold, chronic sweating and headaches.

Another key symptom is alcohol and/or drug abuse. You may notice that your friend or relative is drinking far more than usual. If they already had an unhealthy relationship with drink and drugs, you may see this dramatically worsen.

PTSD can lead to the misuse of alcohol and drugs.
Photo:
www.istockphoto.com

It is hardly surprising that those suffering from anxiety, fear and helplessness might turn to anything that temporarily numbs the cause of their problem. However, a short-term coping strategy can lead to a longer term problem further down the line.

How can PTSD be helped

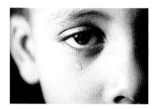

Children are just as vulnerable as adults.
Photo:
www.istockphoto.com

There are a number of things you can do to try and lessen the emotional strain, but be patient as it may take many weeks before you feel back to your normal self. Initially take each day as it comes. Try to do things that make you feel safe and secure. As soon as you can, get back to your usual routine, return to work or in the case of children, encourage them to go back to school. At the same time make an effort to spend time with family and friends and don't hide away. A healthy diet and exercise are also important, but build time into your day for rest and relaxation.

It is fairly common for people with post-traumatic stress not to want to talk about the event. This may help initially, but if you are going to resolve your feelings and emotions in the long-term you are eventually going to have to open up and talk to someone. If you find this difficult, because the people around you weren't there, or you don't feel they would understand, perhaps talk it through with others who were there. If this doesn't work it may be sensible to talk to your doctor.

Children and young people

Children and young people are just as likely to be affected by PTSD as adults. You may notice that they are unsettled, or more aggressive or fearful. They may be more clingy or demanding than usual. Children may repetitively replay the event in the form of games, sometimes aggressively. These are normal reactions and you should notice that over time they gradually reduce. Help them by providing reassurance and support. Just like adults, children cope surprisingly well, and usually come through the experience without any undue long term problems.

Things family and friends can do to help

As a friend, or member of the family, your primary role is to be there for the person and to provide support. Encourage them to talk and then allow them to talk; don't interrupt the flow, or butt in with your own experiences, simply give them time to tell their own story. Just listen.

Support from your friends and family is important.
Photo:
www.istockphoto.com

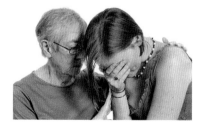

Watch out for any changes in their behaviour. If you are a work colleague note alterations in their work patterns; lateness or excessive or unusual sick leave. You may see changes in personality such as being more irritable, angry, tearful or depressed and showing a general lack of interest.

These behaviours usually settle down after a period of about six weeks, as the person starts to come to terms with their experiences and returns to being their normal self. During this time you need to be as supportive and tolerant as possible. Don't try to empathise or pretend you know how they feel – you don't! And the age old mantra of 'just pull yourself together!' will probably do more harm than good.

Diagnosing PTSD

Not everyone needs professional help to recover from their traumatic experience. Recovery depends on a number of things, including the type and severity of the traumatic experience, your reaction to it, your previous life experiences, your way of coping and the support network you have around you. However, if your symptoms are particularly severe, or after six weeks you do not appear to be getting better, or your symptoms are getting worse, then it might be advisable to visit your doctor for guidance.

Treatment options

Once diagnosed with PTSD you will be guided towards the most appropriate treatment. If only a few weeks have passed since the traumatic event took place, or your symptoms are relatively mild, it may be decided that a period of 'watchful waiting' is advised. In simple terms, you will be closely monitored to see if things get better or worse.

If treatment is recommended the initial approach is usually 'talking treatments' – simply talking through the event. This could be with a counsellor, psychotherapist or psychologist. Other treatments involve teaching you to change the negative thoughts, working through your experience and regaining control of your fears and anxieties. Another treatment called eye movement desensitisation and reprocessing (EMDR) can also be used to help your brain 'sort out' or 'process' your flashbacks in order to come to terms with the event and reduce the level of stress you are experiencing.

Working through your traumatic event will mean having to confront some incredibly uncomfortable and sometimes distressing emotions.

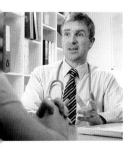

Your doctor may be able to advise you on the best form of treatment.
Photo:
www.istockphoto.com

REAL
LIFE
STORY

Traumatic event

(Neil was climbing with his brother when his traumatic event took place. While down climbing a descent gully his brother slipped and fell. He subsequently died of his injuries.)

For months I wasn't able to get the images of what happened out of my head. I didn't want to talk about it, I didn't want to think about or be reminded of it. I just wanted to get on with my life, as if nothing had actually happened. It felt like my world had been smashed into millions of little tiny pieces. Nothing seemed to be the same; my world no longer seemed to make sense. Even the simplest things like driving the car or shopping were just too much for me. I couldn't cope. It was like all those things that I had learned had simply been erased, deleted. The person that was me seemed gone.

I'd try and distract myself. Take the dog out for a walk or the kids to the park. But the thoughts and feelings wouldn't leave me alone. It felt as if what I had experienced had actually become a permanent part of me. Every day bits of it were happening all over again. I wanted to put it all behind me and move on with my life, but it was as if what I had experienced wouldn't let me. It held me there in that horrific moment in time.

My days, and nights, were periodically filled with horrific reminders of what had happen. It was always there, constantly. I actually dreaded going to sleep at nights; I'd make excuses, do anything to avoid going to bed. Sleep never came easy. I was being haunted. My nightmares were so real; I was there again. Reliving it. The smells, the emotions were unbelievably real. I would wake up crying, real gulping sobs, totally distraught and exhausted. Even when I woke, it took me a while before I realised it was just a dream.

I couldn't move forward; I couldn't get away from the nightmares and flashbacks. I was trapped. It really felt like I was going nuts. I couldn't concentrate on anything and I was always angry for no real reason.

It was my wife who suggested I got professional help. I'd been like this for months and she was struggling to cope with my behaviour. She went to see her doctor and explained what had been going on and he suggested I made an appointment to see him. So I did and he recommended a referral to a therapist. I really did think at this stage that I was going mad. But she helped me to work through what was happening.   ...

I'd describe my treatment as if I had in front of me the pieces of an enormous smashed vase that I was trying to put back together again. Through my treatment I started to find pieces that fitted together. At first it was only a few bits but over time I started to see the bigger picture, I could see what I was trying to achieve. Yes, ok, there were times when I felt I was going backwards, when bits of the vase didn't feel like they belonged anywhere. And yes, at times I wanted to just give up. But I'd invested so much time, energy and emotion to get where I was, I just couldn't throw the towel in. If nothing else, I owed it to my wife and kids.

It took well over a year to get to where I am today. Where am I? I am in control. I'll never be able to forget what happened that day, but the experience has left me far more understanding, forgiving and even tolerant than I ever was before.

Neil

When will I get better?

That is a difficult question to answer; every person is different. What is understood is that it will take time, so you have to be patient. Understanding how traumatic events affect you and being aware of what you can do to help yourself, will hopefully lead you onto the path of recovery. When you can think and talk about the event without becoming upset or distressed and the experience no longer dogs your every waking moment, that's when you have come to terms with your experience.

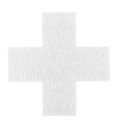

18. MULTIPLE CASUALTY INCIDENTS: TRIAGE

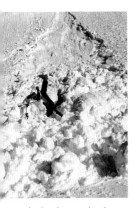

Avalanche – a classic
multiple casualty situation.
Photo: Martin Chester

In an urban environment the emergency services would take control of a multiple casualty accident – normally referred to as a 'major incident'. However, in the remote setting the rescue services could be several hours away; therefore you will need to do what you can, with whatever you have to hand, until that help arrives.

Fortunately the vast majority of incidents in remote locations involve only one casualty. However certain types of accidents can lead to a situation with two or more casualties.

The general approach to multiple casualties is to try to do the most you can for as many people as possible. This involves prioritising which casualties require assistance immediately and identifying those in less need. This process is usually referred to as 'triage', which is a French word meaning 'to sort'. Your initial task therefore will be to sort through the casualties and **prioritise** their treatment and evacuation.

The Triage Categories

Priority 1   Colour: Red – Immediate help and evacuation needed.

Priority 2   Colour: Yellow – Injured whose evacuation can be delayed.

Priority 3   Colour: Green – Walking wounded; the least urgent cases.

Dead   Colour: White – Those beyond help.

Multiple casualty assessment

The following is a guide towards carrying out a rapid triage assessment of multiple casualties. In reality you are unlikely to have to deal with more than one or two. However this assessment covers what to do if you come across the worst case scenario with many casualties.

1. Assess the scene for **danger** before you approach and task someone to summon help as soon as possible. If there are bystanders around, try to recruit them to help.

   > Be very clear about who you ask to get help. Point at someone and task them directly to dial 999/112, ask for police then request mountain rescue. Tell them to come and find you when they have done this. The rescue services will need to know; what type of accident (i.e. avalanche, light aircraft crash, etc.), the location (preferably a grid reference), the access to the incident site, if there are any potential hazards and an approximate number of casualties.

2. Choose a safe area away from the accident scene as a congregation point. Shout loudly for all those who are able to walk to make their way over to this location. If possible ask someone to do this for you and give them the responsibility for monitoring the group. If available provide a group shelter. These are the least urgent casualties and they are given the category of Priority 3 known as the walking wounded.

   > In a mass casualty situation this group often tends to be the largest. It is useful for the person in charge to record each casualty's name, age and undertake a quick SAMPLE assessment (see page 23, Dealing with a Conscious Casualty). Those with minor injuries can be used to perform basic first aid on others if directed.

3. Make your way to the 'quiet' motionless casualties, open their airway and check if they are breathing. If they are **not** breathing they are categorised as **dead** and are beyond help. You must leave them and move on to the next casualty.

   > This sounds rather brutal but remember the aim of triage is to 'do the most for the most' and wasting time on this casualty may result in someone who could have been saved from dying.

4. If the casualty is breathing, quickly count the number of breaths (count breathing for 15 seconds then multiply by 4): if the casualty is breathing less than 10 or more than 30 times in a minute they are classed as **Priority 1**.

If this casualty is breathing rapidly – twice as fast as you – then it is possible they are in blood loss shock. If there is an obvious bleed you could task a bystander, or one of your walking wounded, to apply pressure over any significant external bleed and raise the legs.

5. If the casualty is breathing normally (between 10 and 30 breaths a minute) take a pulse at the neck (count the pulse for 15 seconds then multiply by 4). If the pulse is over 120 beats per minute this casualty is a **Priority 1** and if less than 120 beats per minute they are Priority 2.

If you are not confident taking a pulse you can substitute this with a capillary refill test (CRT) on the torso of the casualty (top of the breast bone). Push down on the skin for 5 seconds then release, the skin should look pale; the area should normally refill in about 2 seconds. If it takes more than 2 seconds then this casualty is a 'priority 1', or if less than 2 seconds they are a 'priority 2'. Capillary refill tests done on the finger nails will probably be delayed because the casualty will be cold; by testing on the torso you stand a better chance of a more accurate result.

Some points to note

It is very tempting, as you make your way around an accident site, to start getting involved with the first aid; however your initial task is to rapidly go round all casualties and sort out who is in most need of assistance. It may be possible for the casualty to treat themselves with some direction and guidance; alternatively you can instruct a bystander or one of the walking wounded to do some basic first aid. It is surprising what people can do with a little coaching. Remember only when those casualties in the highest category of 'Priority 1' have been looked after and treated, should those in the lower categories be given treatment.

This triage sieve is designed for adults and is not suitable for use on children due to the specific breathing rates used.

Summary

Triage is a very dynamic process and casualties do not necessarily remain in one level of priority and stay there throughout the incident; for example a less urgent walking wounded casualty 'Priority 3' can deteriorate becoming a '**Priority 1**' and in need of immediate treatment and evacuation. You will need to constantly re-assess. When the rescue services arrive they will take over and probably perform their own triage assessment. However giving a clear hand over – with as much information as possible – will make their task much easier.

It is unlikely that you will remember the triage sieve, so it is suggested that you transfer the information onto a small 'prompt card' which you can waterproof and store in your outdoor first aid kit.

The triage sieve

Can they walk?	YES	**Priority 3**
	NO	
If quiet open airway breathing?	NO	**Dead**
	YES	
Count breathing under 10 or over 20 breaths per min?	YES	**Priority 1**
	Over 120 pulse (CRT* longer than 2 secs)	
	NO	
Check circulation take a pulse	**Under 120 pulse (CRT 2 secs or less)**	**Priority 2**

*Capillary refill test on the torso.

GLOSSARY

ABCs The primary survey; stands for **A**irway, **B**reathing and **C**irculation.

Abdomen The body cavity that contains the stomach, intestines, liver, spleen and pancreas. Also referred to as the belly.

Abrasion Damage to the surface of the skin from rubbing or scraping across a rough surface.

Agonal gasps Occasional strange, gasping noises that occur when the heart has stopped; is an indicator to start CPR.

Airway The passage by which air enters and leaves the lungs.

Alert A conscious casualty who spontaneously opens their eyes when you approach, speaks clearly, responds to questions, and is aware of and reacts to their environment.

Allergen Something that causes an allergic reaction.

Anaphylactic shock A rapidly progressing, life-threatening allergic reaction.

Antihistamines Drugs used to treat allergic reactions.

Artery A blood vessel that carries blood away from the heart.

Asthma A condition of the airways causing swelling of the tubes inside the lungs and build-up of mucus causing them to narrow. This leads to breathing difficulties.

Auto-injector A medical device used to deliver a single dose of a drug, mainly by a spring loaded injection into the skin.

Automated External Defibrillator (AED) A portable device that can be attached to a casualty who is not breathing. If a shockable heart rhythm is detected the machine will send an electrical current (defibrillation) through the heart allowing it to re-establish an effective rhythm.

AVPU A scale used to measure and record a casualty's level of response; stands for **A**lert, casualty responding to **V**oice, **P**ain or **U**nresponsive.

Basic life support Emergency treatment – cardiopulmonary resuscitation (CPR) – given until more specific medical treatment can begin.

Blunt injury An injury produced by a blunt object or force, in which the skin is not broken.

Capillary refill test (CRT) A test that evaluates the circulation by squeezing the blood from the area (such as skin or nail bed) then watching the speed of its return after releasing the pressure.

Cardiac arrest The sudden stopping of the heart's ability to pump.

Cardiopulmonary resuscitation (CPR) An emergency procedure on a casualty who is not breathing, involving compressing the chest and breathing for the casualty.

Casualty The term used to describe a person who is in need of first aid.

Casualty report form A form that details the casualty's condition and further observations to assist in the casualty assessment and 'hand over' to further medical assistance.

Cerebral Relating to the brain.

Cervical spine The part of the spine that makes up the neck.

Clot A thick, coagulated mass or lump of blood.

Coma A state of deep, often long-lasting unconsciousness.

Concussion A mild injury to the brain from an impact to the head.

Contamination The presence of organisms or foreign bodies such as dirt, grass or manure.

Contraindication A specific situation in which a drug should NOT be used, because it may be harmful to the casualty.

Core The central, innermost part of anything. In its basic context the core is the body minus the arms and legs (i.e. including the heart, lungs, liver and other vital organs).

Crepitus A grinding noise/sensation caused by broken bone ends rubbing together.

Cyanosis A bluish/grey skin colour caused by a lack of oxygen in the body.

Diabetes An inability to regulate the body's blood glucose levels.

Diaphragm A dome of muscle that sits underneath the lungs and assists in breathing.

Dilated Expanded or widened.

Dislocation The temporary displacement of a bone from its normal position; usually a joint.

Diuretics Medication that reduces the amount of fluid in the body by increasing urine output.

Drowning Someone who has been under the surface of the water (or liquid) and experiences breathing impairment.

Ectopic pregnancy A pregnancy that develops outside of the womb; usually in the Fallopian tube.

Epilepsy A common condition in which a person has recurrent seizures (also referred to as a fit or convulsion).

Epinephrine Also known as adrenaline; a hormone which can be produced by the body or administered as a drug. This is the drug used to treat anaphylaxis.

Evacuate Removing the casualty from the remote setting by either one's own efforts or through the rescue services.

Face shield A device used when giving rescue breaths to a casualty who has stopped breathing which protects the user from cross infections.

FAST A method of assessing a casualty whom you suspect has had a stroke. Face, Arms, Speech, Time to dial 999/112.

Flail chest When enough ribs are broken to threaten the rigidity of the chest.

Fracture A break in a bone.

Frostbite   Freezing of the extremity resulting in tissue damage (can be mild or deep).

Frostnip   Superficial cooling of the extremity without tissue damage.

Full thickness burn   A deep burn affecting all layers of the skin and can include muscle, bone and internal organs.

Hyper arousal   The fight-or-flight response in which the casualty is always on alert, has trouble sleeping, is irritable, has difficulty concentrating, and displays an exaggerated startle response.

Hyperglycaemia   Abnormally high blood sugar (glucose) levels.

Hyperthermia   An elevated core body temperature causing overheating.

Hyperventilation   Breathing faster or deeper than normal. Sometimes referred to as 'over breathing'.

Hypoglycaemia   Abnormally low blood sugar (glucose) levels.

Hypothermia   A condition where the core body temperature falls below 35°C usually from prolonged exposure to cool or freezing temperatures.

Initial assessment   This is the first part of your remote setting casualty assessment in which you make an initial check for the level of response (AVPU) and complete your primary survey (ABCs).

Irrigation   To wash out a wound with water.

Jaw thrust   A method of opening the airway in which there is no movement of the neck; used in the unconscious casualty whom you suspect has a spinal injury.

Laceration   A rough, jagged tear-like wound.

Level of Response   An assessment of whether a casualty is conscious or unconscious through the use of the AVPU scale.

Ligaments   Fibrous tissue that connects bones to bones.

Log roll   A method of turning a casualty from a position on their back when you suspect a spinal injury. Can be used to assess for injuries or to place into a safe airway position.

Mechanisms of injury   The way in which the injury occurred and the forces involved in the accident.

Mucus   A thick slimy fluid produced by membranes lining certain organs in the body.

Nausea   An unpleasant feeling that often leads to vomiting.

Neutral position   Head, neck and spine are all aligned in a straight line.

Open fracture   Any break in a bone in which the overlying skin has been broken.

Palpate   Examine by touch.

Panda eyes   Bruising under the eyes which may indicate a skull fracture.

Paralysis   The loss of movement and/or feeling.

Partial thickness burn   A burn that causes redness and clear blisters to form.

Post traumatic stress disorder (PTSD)   An anxiety disorder that occurs after experiencing a traumatic event.

Primary survey   The ABCs of first aid (**A**irway, **B**reathing, **C**irculation).

Pulse   The wave of pressure created by the beat of the heart down the arteries.

Pupil The circular opening in the centre of the iris (coloured part of the eye) that allows light into the back of the eye.

Respiratory arrest Breathing has stopped.

RICE Treatment for soft tissue injuries; stands for **R**est, **I**ce **C**ompression, and **E**levation.

Safe airway position (Also known as the recovery position.) This is **any** position where the mouth is lower than the back of the throat, avoiding suffocation from obstruction of the airway by the tongue and/or drowning in vomit or blood.

SAMPLE A mnemonic to help the first aider remember how to approach the secondary survey; **S**igns and symptoms, **A**llergies, **M**edications, **P**revious medical history, **L**ast meal, **E**vents (what happened).

Secondary survey Part of the remote casualty assessment which involves dealing with the injury or medical conditions and if necessary undertaking a full head-to-toe examination of the casualty.

Seizure (Also referred to as a fit or convulsion.) Random chaotic electrical bursts of activity in the brain.

Sign An objective finding that can be seen, heard, smelt or measured (e.g. a skin rash).

Spinal cord An extension of the brain consisting of millions of nerves which allow the brain and the muscles to communicate. It sits in the spinal canal and is protected in fluid and surrounded by the spinal column.

Spine Also known as backbone and consists of the vertebra bones and the discs in between.

Splint A rigid device used to immobilise a fracture.

Status epilepticus A continuous seizure lasting for 30 minutes or more which is potentially life-threatening.

Superficial burn Reddening of the surface of the skin.

Symptoms A subjective finding that the casualty feels and expresses (e.g. a casualty feeling nauseous).

Tendons A tough rope-like fibrous tissue that attaches muscles to bone.

Tenting When the skin is stretched over a broken bone or dislocation. The stretched skin appears taught and white.

Tetanus This is a serious bacterial illness. The bacteria live in dust, soil, saliva and manure, and usually enter the body through an open wound on the skin.

Tourniquet A last-resort method of controlling catastrophic life-threatening external bleeding.

Triage The process of sorting multiple casualties to prioritise their need for immediate treatment and speed of evacuation.

Unresponsive The unconscious casualty who does not respond to voice or pain stimulus.

Vertebrae The bones that make up the spinal column.

Vital signs The key signs used to evaluate a casualty's overall condition and includes breathing, pulse, level of response, temperature and skin colour.

INDEX